Praise for *Your Extraordinary Mind*

"From living with his world-famous father to spending his teenage years as a Deadhead, Zach Leary was destined to wrestle the angel of psychedelia. *Your Extraordinary Mind* contains an outstandingly well-informed and multi-perspectival view on sacred substances, as well as the best advice on their use, impact, promise, and perils. In this heartful book about how we can get the most out of our consciousness, Zach Leary joins the wisest of psychedelic cultural voices."

ALEX GREY AND ALLYSON GREY
visionary artist cofounders of Chapel of Sacred Mirrors

"Excellent, helpful, knowledgeable, and heartfelt. Zach Leary offers us a thorough and wise guide to skillfully understand, navigate, and use the power of psychedelics and the gifts of sacred medicine."

JACK KORNFIELD
author of *A Path with Heart*

"Zach Leary, with his front-row seat to the story of psychedelics in America, takes you on a fantastic journey, exploring the history and science of psychedelics and their implications for consciousness studies; death, dying, and grief; spirituality; and other landscapes of human experience. And he does so with warmth and compassion."

ANTHONY P. BOSSIS, PHD
New York University School of Medicine

YOUR EXTRAORDINARY MIND

YOUR EXTRAORDINARY MIND

Psychedelics in the 21st Century and How to Use Them

ZACH LEARY

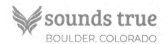

sounds true
BOULDER. COLORADO

Sounds True
Boulder, CO

The information in this book seeks to provide an understanding of the author's personal experiences with psychedelics and is intended for general information purposes only. It is not meant to take the place of diagnosis and treatment by a qualified medical practitioner or therapist and does not represent advocacy for illegal activities. It is a criminal offense in the United States and in many other countries, punishable by imprisonment and/or fines, to manufacture, possess, or supply some of the substances mentioned, except in connection with government-sanctioned research. This information is not intended to encourage you to break the law and no attempt should be made to use these substances for any purpose except in a capacity that is legally sanctioned on a state or federal level. The author and publisher expressly disclaim any liability, loss, or risk, personal or otherwise, that is incurred as a consequence, directly or indirectly, of the contents of this book. Any application of the material set forth in the following pages is at the reader's discretion and is their sole responsibility.

Some names and identifying details have been changed to protect the privacy of individuals.

Published 2025

Cover and jacket design by Jennifer Miles
Book design by Scribe Inc.

Printed in Canada

BK06523

Library of Congress Cataloging-in-Publication Data

Names: Leary, Zach, author.
Title: Your extraordinary mind : psychedelics in the 21st century and how to use them / Zach Leary.
Description: Boulder, CO : Sounds True, 2025. | Includes index.
Identifiers: LCCN 2024041350 (print) | LCCN 2024041351 (ebook) | ISBN 9781683649939 (trade paperback) | ISBN 9781683649946 (ebook)
Subjects: LCSH: Hallucinogenic drugs. | Hallucinogenic drugs--Therapeutic use.
Classification: LCC RM324.8 .L43 2025 (print) | LCC RM324.8 (ebook) | DDC 615.7/883--dc23/eng/20250111
LC record available at https://lccn.loc.gov/2024041350
LC ebook record available at https://lccn.loc.gov/2024041351

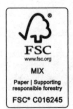

FSC
www.fsc.org
MIX
Paper | Supporting
responsible forestry
FSC® C016245

To Timmy for lighting the flame
. . . and to Ram Dass for keeping the flame lit

And to Heather, my beloved and partner whose love
and support made this book come to life

Contents

Introduction

Every psychedelic trip has its beginnings. For some people, it's setting an intention for what they hope to contemplate during their experience—that thirst for a transcendental connection that may appear, however fleeting. For those suffering from mental health disorders, their journey may begin with the suggestion that there is another route to ease their suffering. For the mystically inclined, it may be that warm hug when the medicine starts to kick in and the unsettling satisfaction of knowing that, for the next few hours, they will be greeted with insight into the idea that whatever they think reality is, it's not. There are so many unique and varied reasons why someone might want to set forth on the ancient yet modernly relevant practice of using psychedelic plants and medicines.

Just as there are many reasons why people may want to use psychedelics today, there are many origins and histories of these substances and their culture. As we explore the colorful tapestries within these mind-expanding plants and chemicals, we begin to see some historical commonalities that anyone interested in using psychedelics should take the time to understand before embarking on their discovery of their mind's inner workings.

My life is a living example of this sequence of events. I grew up in a household so full of psychedelic lore that my childhood mind vibrated with an unwavering curiosity about what these drugs were all about and why the man who was raising me was so famous. Contrary to popular opinion, when I first considered the idea of using psychedelics at age fifteen, my parents were not okay with me becoming a teenage psychonaut, aka a psychedelic explorer. I was following the Grateful Dead around the country, and there was no way I could "just say no." My father sat me down and said plainly, "Zach, LSD is a very powerful tool, and you have to know that your brain is not fully developed yet. I strongly encourage you to wait until you're older before taking it."

Of course I didn't. Even so, my father's cautionary advice took hold in my mind, and I became a very cautious and deliberate young acid head who tried to make sure the principles of "set and setting" were adhered to for every trip I went on. "Set" is the voyager's mindset and inner condition, and "setting" is the environment in which you surround yourself while on the drug.

Looking back on those days, now thirty-five years ago, a huge part of my curiosity was rooted in the cultural tradition I was surrounded by. Twentieth-century psychedelic luminaries like Timothy Leary, Ram Dass, John C. Lilly, Terence McKenna, and Dr. Oz Janiger were all fixtures in my home, and that, combined with the seductive power of the Dead's scene, made me feel like I was being lured into a hero's journey that I was yet to fully understand, but I sure as hell was going to try.

The tales of the modern explorers of consciousness have taken on an almost folklorish status: wild-eyed modern mystics trekking into the jungles of South America seeking the elusive Ayahuasca vine, brilliant yet prickly Harvard professors challenging the very institutions that they are part of by preaching the power of LSD to a younger generation, or a young psychology student so enamored with the therapeutic potential of MDMA that he set forth on a thirty-year odyssey to tell the world all about it.

These are great stories to tell and for you to understand. It's important to understand the history of psychedelics in America because it can help make you more cautious and knowledgeable on the quest that you may or may not undertake. This book is not solely about psychedelic culture and its storied history. It's also about creating an instructional road map that allows the end user to find a symbiotic relationship with psychedelic drugs that has long-lasting, positive effects on their life, both spiritually and psychologically. This is accomplished through becoming educated about the specific compounds, having a very solid plan for set and setting, and paying extra care to what we now refer to simply as "integration," or the work that comes after the journey.

Over the course of the last several years, as psychedelics have become more palatable within our culture and accepted within therapeutic circles, I've started to notice a need to create an accessible resource for safe and effective psychedelic use that is appropriate for all variations of seekers, ranging from the spiritually curious to the therapist who is planning on introducing them as a healing method into their client-centered practice.

Being Timothy Leary's son and Ram Dass's student makes for strange bedfellows. I've been able to find a union of Timothy's passion for the individual mandate to control one's mind and to "trust one's nervous system." Ram Dass's path of cultivating the heart into a wellspring of unconditional love and compassion may seem like a very different path than Leary's, and perhaps it is, but I find there to be a synergistic relationship that is necessary to go forth on the spiritual path. Through the work I've done on myself and in formal study with Ram Dass in America and around the world (India mostly), I've come to learn that there is a deep hunger for a new approach to set and setting, and for young people who are new to this method to get acquainted with the histories of these compounds. And finally, there is a dire need for helping people get more clarity about what to do after the journey, aka "integration."

Turning insight into action that results in these drugs having a more sustained effect on one's life rather than feeling the need to keep chasing the peak experience is something I'm very passionate about. Later on in the book, you'll find some question sets and recommendations on how this can be achieved.

When I started working with others as their psychedelic guide and coach, I began to notice a constant reoccurring sentiment: growth isn't about becoming someone new; it's about uncovering the authenticity of one's inner self that's been there all along. For many reasons, getting in touch with the most authentic expression of our truest selves gets lost. Psychedelic exploration and the integration process that comes afterward are a wonderful acceleration for that rediscovery. Your extraordinary mind can get burst wide open. There you can discover unknown parts of yourself that can lead to a better understanding of who you are and perhaps even a deeper connection to the entirety of your humanity—namely, the cultivation of the heart.

In the 1960s, as fantastic as they were, psychedelics ultimately fell into a pattern of reckless use. It's important that we recognize where the road map for psychedelic use in the '60s went wrong and how we can learn from those mistakes to make a better future for the current psychedelic movement. By educating our culture about the profound power and potential risks of psychedelics, we can help reduce the number of bad trips and psychotic breaks and present the public with the cold, hard fact that not all psychedelics are for all people. Not everyone is cut out to be an explorer of their minds in this way. Those who are, however, are better served if they are equipped with a solid methodology on how to use psychedelic drugs successfully, which includes safety protocols, spiritual guidelines, risk-versus-reward assessment, and access to pure chemical compounds that won't damage their bodies. Essentially, this is a harm-reduction approach to psychedelic use.

We are at a fantastic crossroads filled with great promise, but we are also at risk of keeping the movement in the hands of labs and medical professionals. I don't condone indiscriminate use of any drug, especially in the hands of young people who are at risk of using powerful mind/soul-altering psychotropics in an unstructured and dangerous way. Because of this, it's important that we continue to learn from the medical research about the safe use of psychedelics to treat mental health conditions. That does not mean that we can altogether abandon the notion of cognitive liberty, aka the freedom to change one's consciousness as they see fit.

I've become fixated on the reasons why people want to use psychedelic drugs and, subsequently, how they might take that experience and integrate it into their lives for years to come. Some say the psychedelic experience is too vast and unconventional to be reduced into language that can affect its daily relationship with consciousness. While I do resonate with Terence McKenna's chestnut, "There is a space beyond language, it's just so damn hard to talk about," I also subscribe to the idea that the psychedelic experience can be woven into one's heart, soul, healing, and thus daily living practice. I believe we can distill the mind-blowing, previously indescribable psychedelic experience, into a focused spiritual method that can help people in their daily lives.

This book explores what that method looks like and shares stories around my life, my personal psychedelic experiences, my observations as a psychedelic facilitator, and commentaries on the current psychedelic renaissance. There are also elements that serve as a guide manual (of sorts) for the individual who wants to plot their own course for successful healing, growth, and self-inquiry. This book is just the beginning of a larger conversation that I hope will extend into the psychedelic community at large and to whoever is seeking the promise of a better quality of life.

So before we get into the meat and potatoes of how psychedelics can be used safely, effectively, and with a purpose that goes beyond the limitations of the human condition and our so-called medical establishment, I want to briefly recount some of the history of how we got to this moment in time—a place that is now fondly referred to as the psychedelic renaissance.

Technically speaking, the word "renaissance" is defined as "a revival or renewed interest in something." While it's true that the current fervor of interest in psychedelics is the most active that it's ever been since the 1960s, it is also vital to point out that psychedelics have never been adopted in the West as a method for serious healing and spiritual growth without ambiguity, controversy, and propaganda. The '60s were a blip that showed us what's possible, but sadly it didn't last.

However, Indigenous cultures have long been incorporating psyche-delic use as a core part of their cultures and healing paradigms.

It's my deepest wish that today's world continues to investigate the vast potential of psychedelic drugs and medicines, and lands on the conclusion that they are just as valid a methodology for the better-ment of human evolution as anything else we've tried.

The History of Psychedelics: The Twentieth-Century Rebirth

In May 1961, after embarking on his first psilocybin journey, my father Timothy Leary proclaimed with an awestruck sense of trans-formation, "I learned more about psychology in the five hours after taking these mushrooms than in the preceding fifteen years of study-ing and doing research in psychology."

Leary's colleague and psychonautic cohort Richard Alpert (later known as Ram Dass), mesmerized after hearing of Timothy's mush-room experience, decided to go on his own inaugural psilocybin journey a few months later. He recalled "the first encounter" with poetic reflection: "I knew myself was gone, still there was something in me that was watching this whole process disappear. There was what I at the time was calling a scanning device or a point of awareness; something in there that had no reference to body; no reference to personality; no reference to any of my social roles, and yet there it was, clear and lucid and watching the whole thing and just, you know, watching it all happen."

Leary's and Alpert's journeys happened in the context of a perfect storm of cultural, political, and scientific advancement that became one of the great cultural revolutions in mankind's history: the 1960s. Some may look back on them now as just thoughtful neo-spiritual recollections of a psychedelic experience, but in 1961, this was a very big deal for two Harvard professors to proclaim. Everything about Western culture and society was about to change.

Not only did the Western world become aware of the profound power of psychedelic drugs thanks to research at Harvard and Ken

Kesey's now legendary "Acid Tests," but simultaneously our day-to-day life as a society was being led by a youth-driven kaleidoscope of social activism, avant-garde rock music, daring fashions, civil and women's rights, and countless other movements that would have been unrecognizable to the 1950s establishment. As wise old Timothy once said, "In order to understand the 1960s, you first must understand the 1950s."

It suddenly became permissible to question the draconian restrictions of your parents' generation by expanding your field of vision to think for yourself, worship new gods or no gods at all, study new fields of artistic expression, have premarital sex, try new fashion, and follow your heart instead of following the worker bee tradition. This scared the establishment because it laid the foundation for the introduction of non-Christian values into the Western zeitgeist that began the process of piercing the veil of the patriarchal and capitalist systems that ruled the day. The very concept of perceiving your consciousness in an entirely new way as a result of using newfound drugs like LSD and smoking cannabis couldn't help but create a subculture of millions who were quick to question authority and give rise to an Aquarian Age.

Even though psychedelic drugs felt new to people trying them for the first time in the 1960s, the reality is they weren't actually new at all. The practice of gathering as a community in ceremony around a psychedelic sacrament can be found in Indigenous cultures dating back thousands of years through the present. There is strong archeological evidence that places the use of magic mushrooms as far away as ancient Siberia and the use of ergot in the ritual celebrations of ancient Greece, known as the Eleusinian Mysteries.

Prior to 1961 (when Leary and Alpert did their first mushroom trip) the proliferation of psychedelics gained a lot of traction in the 1950s, as icons like Aldous Huxley encountered the magical properties of mescaline thanks to Dr. Humphry Osmond, the great psychotherapist who coined the term "psychedelic," which translates to "mind manifesting."

Still, before the counterculture of the '60s took hold, the acceptance of psychedelics on a wide level could only be seen within the traditions of Indigenous cultures that used them (and still do) as methods for healing, celebration, and deep inner knowing. Notably, the Shipibo people of Peru and their healers use Ayahuasca to induce mystical revelations, and the Aztecs found magic mushrooms to be so spiritually potent that they named them Teonanácatl, aka "the flesh of the Gods." The use of psilocybin mushrooms within regions of Mexico, like Cuernavaca, revolve around tribal rituals infused with hints of Catholic saints and local traditions—both of which center around the understanding that mysticism is not separate from our waking reality, that it is merely another layer of one persistent reality. These wisdom seekers know that God is everywhere and in everything, and that in order to lead a more holistic life, you must recognize this non-duality.

In the modern Western world, these practices of entheogenic celebrations and ritual became all but lost. There are some accounts of colonists coming across Indigenous use of Ayahuasca and magic mushrooms, but it seems none of those sightings struck enough curiosity to bring them back to their homelands.

It wasn't until 1954 that the book *The Doors of Perception* by Aldous Huxley became the first "mainstream" account of how psychedelics can offer a different relationship to one's own mystical landscape found within the heart and mind. Huxley became acutely aware that humans didn't have to search for external doorways to achieve spiritual enlightenment, instead suggesting it was within us all along.

He reflects on his own use of mescaline by writing, "The man who comes back through the Door in the Wall will never be quite the same as the man who went out. He will be wiser but less sure, happier but less self-satisfied, humbler in acknowledging his ignorance yet better equipped to understand the relationship of words to things . . ."

At that time, most of the Western world didn't know much about how Indigenous cultures were using mind-altering plants as sacraments in their rituals. But in 1956, the magazine that was on every coffee table in the '40s and '50s, *LIFE*, ran a story called "Seeking the Magic Mushroom." It's safe to say that R. Gordon Wasson's *LIFE Magazine* account of his travels in Mexico and encounter with curandera María Sabina brought sacred mushroom use into the American household almost overnight. Wasson, with his wife, took *LIFE* readers on a trip to the remote mountains of Mexico, where they spent years documenting the ceremonial use of mushrooms that had "vision giving powers." This was strong stuff for the pages of *LIFE* in the 1950s. The article is incredibly objective and full of rich and curious insights into the potential of these wild fungi and the people who were using them. It's far less full of fear-based propaganda than you might expect considering it was published in 1956.

When Leary and Alpert began their work at Harvard in 1961, there was some cultural precedent, thanks to Huxley and Wasson, and some documented therapeutic use, thanks to Osmond, Janiger, and Hartman. But that didn't mean a major Ivy League institution was ready to blow the doors off traditional psychology just yet. These two outliers, in the role of dutiful Harvard professors, began conducting research into the very nature of consciousness, divinity, cognitive liberty, and the social constructs that flew in the face of conventional society.

The problem was that the Harvard elite had very different ideas for how the departmental rules and regulations for an ethical and responsible psychology department should be run. Those rules, of which many were indeed broken, ultimately appeared to be holding Leary and Alpert back from forging on to the lofty goals they had for revolutionizing the human condition. Sure enough, they both got fired from Harvard in 1963—not for shoddy research but for tales of faculty-student fraternization exposed by an undergraduate reporter for the local Harvard newspaper. They were looking for any reason to fire Leary and Alpert, and that was just a convenient excuse. The impact they were having was simply too much for a very conservative Ivy League institution.

Not to be deterred, they continued their work at Millbrook, an upstate New York estate that was extended to them by the

Mellon-Hitchcock family. What happened there (and at Harvard) set the psychedelic research movement on fire, and the various results have been hotly debated over the last fifty years. Setting aside how you may feel about Timothy Leary personally, his and Alpert's contribution to the early psychedelic canon was one of the elements that spawned the huge cultural changes of the 1960s.

Still, many modern psychedelic voices who are popular in today's movement like to say they are "cleaning up the mess that Leary made" by getting psychedelic research back on track due to Leary's court-jester-like antics. Questions have also been raised on the validity of the research data in his projects, such as the Good Friday and Concord Prison experiments. No matter how good the data was or wasn't, or the profound impact LSD use had on popular culture, the 1960s use of psychedelics helped spawn an unwelcome war on drugs that took down legitimate psychedelic research with it. Timothy Leary became more of a symbol of antidrug hysteria created by Richard Nixon's administration than anything else. He was persecuted and put in prison, escaped from prison, and was locked up again, and through all of that, he held his head high as he continued to live by the mantra "think for yourself and question authority."

Revisiting the War on Drugs

This is true: Leary's antics led him to become a political figure more than anything else, and that took away from the serious work that psychedelics were gaining traction on. What many anti-Leary soldiers conveniently forget is that there is no way any one of us could know what it was like to be in Leary's shoes. More to the point, it's impossible to believe that Richard Nixon would have set aside a place for psychedelics in a research setting had he been given a different data set when he launched the modern War on Drugs. Not a chance.

The War on Drugs was a war against people he didn't like (more on that later), and the counterculture hippy kids who were doing LSD were no exception. Nixon noticed that those kids were the ones burning their draft cards and protesting in the streets for causes like civil rights and women's equality. Psychedelic drugs were collateral damage.

"The first casualty of any war is the truth, and the war on drugs is no exception," said Neil Woods, a former undercover drug officer in the UK who now leads drug reform policies. This couldn't be more true when tracing the history of psychedelics and their effectiveness, and juxtaposing it against their place in the War on Drugs. In 1970, no one in the federal government cared about their breakthrough potentials, data, or firsthand accounts. The truth didn't matter.

I know firsthand that Timothy Leary never sought to be the leader of any movement or spokesperson for LSD. He did take the role that was offered by the collective and did it with great showbiz flair. At the time, he didn't realize the personal toll he'd have to pay for becoming so infamous. Hunted by the government, thrown in prison, and losing his children all combined to make the rest of Leary's life difficult and full of traumatic wounds that were tough to heal.

But by then LSD was in the hands of millions of people who had very little instruction for how to use it or a road map on what to do after undergoing so many trips. They were armed with little more than a promise that this magical substance could break them free from the confines of their parents' "trip."

The results of some of the vast global recreational LSD use gave us magical, timeless tombs of wonder like "Sgt. Pepper's Lonely Hearts Club Band," the eventuality of Richard Alpert becoming Ram Dass and writing *Be Here Now*, and the lasting magic of cross-sectional communal ceremonial culture like Burning Man and the Grateful Dead. The downsides could be, and have been, argued about endlessly. And they are valid. But to ignore the endless positive cultural contributions that psychedelics have played a part in is absurd.

By 1970, all psychedelic plants and medicines (including cannabis) were Schedule 1 drugs, putting an end to research. So the question remains: who or what slowed down the eventuality of legitimate psychedelic research coming back, and why did it go underground for so many years? Did Leary's (admittedly non-serious) "Tune In, Turn

On, Drop Out" mantra inspire an entire generation to drop out of conventional society and lead the powers that be to crack down on their newfound anti-authoritarian outlook?

Nixon certainly thought so. His racist, anti-counterculture, pro-Vietnam war legislation was more of a scorched-earth approach than it was a calculated dialogue. While trying his best to burn down the uprising, he was fine with taking down psychedelic research along with it. The War on Drugs had officially begun. I seriously doubt that Nixon would have created a different place in our drug laws for psychedelics with or without Leary, Ram Dass, Ken Kesey, and the rest.

The Rebirth of Psychedelic Research

Fast-forward twenty-five years. When the Multidisciplinary Association for Psychedelic Studies (MAPS) started in 1986, founder Rick Doblin made a strategic decision to advance the use of psychedelics by focusing the use of MDMA as a treatment for PTSD by targeting a population that nearly every American agrees is in crisis due to trauma: veterans. This not only was a very effective decision from a therapeutic perspective, but it also was a brilliant move to play considering the support for vets is not a political one, but a moral one. No one could criticize wanting to help veterans.

MAPS was poised straight from the gate to usher in a new dawn of psychedelic research, and in order to do it, the organization had to disassociate itself from the antics of 1960s hippie burnout hysteria. I don't blame Doblin for creating a little distance from the counterculture in order to usher in a new dawn of legitimate psychedelic research. Public perception had to change, and while I don't support that tactic, I do understand it from a political point of view.

It is worth pointing out, without equivocation, that MAPS was on the forefront, battling to make good on its mission statement. MAPS and Lykos (formerly the MAPS Public Benefit Corporation) have taken the lead in manifesting a new dawn of legitimate psychedelic research by trying to be the first to get FDA approval for a psychedelic to be used in conjunction with psychotherapy. At the time of writing this book, MAPS/Lykos completed the phase three clinical trials that would allow MDMA to be prescribed for the treatment of PTSD under the supervision of a therapist. Unfortunately though, the FDA rejected the approval of the Lykos-led submission, ushering in a devastating blow to the legitimate and legal use of psychedelics. Not only did the FDA's rejection of MDMA for the treatment of PTSD affect the vast number of people who could benefit from the therapy, it also slowed down any change in federal policy surrounding the rescheduling of psychedelics as it relates to the War on Drugs. At present, drugs like MDMA are still Schedule 1 narcotics, which means that, according to the federal government, they show no effectiveness for treating mental health. Anyone who has been in the psychedelic community for as long as I have of course knows that this is both absurd and offensive. The long road ahead in getting mainstream psychiatry and organizations like the FDA to accept this ground-breaking modality is long and winding, but I am confident that there will be a path forward that can help save lives and change the fabric of healing.

Thanks to the fire that Leary and Ram Dass started in the '60s, the fantastical and brilliant ramblings of Terence McKenna in the '80s and '90s, and the wonderful scholarly work that people like Rick Doblin, Sasha and Ann Shulgin, Roland Griffiths, Rick Strassman, and many others have done, a new pathway is emerging for how psychedelic drugs can be used by and accepted into the mainstream. As a result of the tireless work that MAPS and many others have done, these drugs now have a legitimate place in the world of psychotherapy, treating PTSD, addiction issues, and a host of other conditions that plague nearly every one of us. It's strange for a pathologically anti-authoritarian person such as myself to have found so much respect for many (certainly not all) in the field of today's academic and medicalized psychedelic movement. I've learned that my energy is best spent in advocating for everyone to have a seat at the ever-expanding psychedelic table. Hanging on to the idea that these mystical compounds have no place in the mainstream doesn't serve anyone.

The studies that MAPS has done with veterans suffering from PTSD, the Johns Hopkins psilocybin divinity project, and the NYU psilocybin palliative care study all show the efficacy that responsible and intentional use of psychedelics can produce when assisting with therapy.

This is all good news, and one aspect that I find so fascinating about some of these current legal clinical trials is the halo effect they have produced. Their success has changed the minds of countless people who otherwise might not have budged in their firm anti-drug stance. For example, far right former Texas governor (and Trump cabinet member) Rick Perry gave one of the opening keynote addresses at the last Psychedelic Science conference in support of treating PTSD in vets with MDMA. Data and personal stories of transformation are very convincing arguments, far more powerful than I could have imagined.

This is real progress, but I'm still convinced that we have a very long way to go. There isn't as much discussion within the psychedelic community around cognitive liberty (being allowed to change our consciousness as we see fit) and ending the War on Drugs as there should be. Yes, there are many efforts to fast-track decriminalization, but most of the bills on the table do so through the lens of psychedelic-assisted therapy and not recreational use.

I can't be hypocritical by dismissing this sort of assisted therapy because I spend much of my time working in this field both with clients and medical professionals, helping curious and desperate people find relief through this method. It's important to remember that it's a marathon and not a sprint; successful medicalization rollouts can lead to changes in personal use as well.

It's a complicated issue with many nuances and arguments both extremely valid and utterly hypocritical. It is my hope that by exploring how psychedelics can be used in the twenty-first century with reverence, safety, and intent that the reader can make up their own mind.

How I Got Here

For the first thirty years of my adult life, I wanted nothing much to do with the psychedelic community. After the death of my father, I struggled tremendously with drug abuse, and when I found recovery, I thought the best thing I could do was create an identity for myself that was as far away from my upbringing as possible. It's not that I just wanted to form my own life, it was also partially a response to the false belief that I had nothing to add to a movement that was largely created by my father—a person who was so extraordinarily blessed with intellect and inspiration.

In that season of life, I had a career as a digital marketer and technology strategist, working on global consumer brands and overseeing the digital presence for internationally successful rock bands. As a result, I spent most of my thirties and early forties going to an office every day from nine to five. It was a very conventional way of life. On the surface, that seemed like pretty good stuff. Stuff that would make my mother proud and could be considered the pinnacle accomplishments of American society. It turned out that path was finding out about who I wasn't, not who I was. Getting as far away from the Leary legacy was an important milestone in my own evolution because it showed me that life can be so rewarding when you try out different roles in order to see which one suits you best and which ones don't fit at all. It's like trying on different clothes in the dharma shop of life.

After about ten years working in the fields of digital marketing and tech strategy, I found that I really wasn't all that good at it. It wasn't because I didn't have the talent or the insight to deliver great work to my clients, it was because my heart was not in it. At around year thirteen, this became obvious, and my world came crashing down. I found myself isolated in a marketing company that I helped cofound and was at tremendous odds with my partner. Deeply saddened, lost, and confused, a great idea hit me: go visit Ram Dass.

In a classic case of identity crisis and feeling like my heart was absent from my life, I rediscovered both my relationship with and passion for Ram Dass. It had been about five years since I last saw him. He had moved to Maui permanently, and I never felt pulled to visit him in his new island abode, not because I didn't want to but because I found myself so ensconced in the corporate facade I had created for myself that spiritual life wasn't a priority. The early influence he had on my life never went away, but the lifestyle of being involved in the "spiritual" community sure did.

I've heard there is a transformation for practitioners that is actually quite common: those that take up yoga (the American asana or posture-based version) can then become inspired to dive deeper into Eastern contemplative practices. The halo effect of the exercise portion of yoga can spark a deeper curiosity. And so it was with me. In 2007, amidst my time at the advertising agency, I started taking regular yoga classes at a place called Sacred Movement in Venice, California. This particular yoga studio featured all the heavy-hitting teachers of the Western yoga explosion in that moment, including Shiva Rea, Saul David Raye, and Mark Whitwell, to name a few. Then in 2008, Saul, in particular, had a profound influence on me. There was just something about his delivery that re-sparked a seeker's curiosity in me. His fusing of Eastern philosophy, kirtan, and Western pragmatism into his vinyasa flow classes was a very welcome counter to the complicated acrobatic and competitive yoga that I was seeing become so popular. His practice was rooted in the heart, self-inquiry, and the quest to discover one's soul. After going to his classes for about six months, a little light started to wake up. It didn't take fully until a couple of years later when I was deep into the tension with my aforementioned business partner.

I began to revisit my Ram Dass book collection, which led to me rediscovering his audio recordings as well. After months of listening to the recordings, reading the books, and immersing myself into the collective works of Ram Dass, it suddenly hit me: "Hey, I know him! I love Ram Dass, and he loves me! Why don't I go see him again?" Saul David Raye became the teacher who appeared at the right time in the right space and when I was able to receive it. The student was suddenly ready. To this day I am so grateful for Saul for sparking my spiritual heart and sending me on a path that eventually led me back to Ram Dass.

So, myself and my brilliant artist friend, light photographer Dean Chamberlain, booked a flight and went to visit Ram Dass on the island of Maui. On the second morning there, at around 5:30 a.m., I got up and decided to go meditate in the living room. Because of jet lag, I was the first one up. I sat there in the living room surrounded by pictures of Ram Dass's guru Neem Karoli Baba, Hanuman, and countless other spiritual artifacts. I suddenly fell into a deep trance.

At first the trance felt joyful, introspective, and full of the qualities that told me I was exactly in the right place. Twenty minutes later, things began to change. A deep sorrow fell over for me, a sadness even. I was hit with an image of myself at age eighty as a man who never lived the life he wanted. A man who sacrificed his own sense of fulfillment for the sake of convenience. It was a glimpse into a tragic figure, and everything in me cried out, "Please don't let that be me, God! Please don't let that be me! What can I do about it?"

In that moment, I realized that if I kept leading the life I was living, I would feel empty and have no true satisfaction in the gift of my incarnation. Even in the best moments of my corporate marketing career, no matter how good they were, there was always this underlying feeling that I was executing someone else's vision. I really had no interest in being a part of that formulaic approach to manifesting the American dream. This isn't to say that I didn't learn a lot while working on accounts like Apple, U2, Depeche Mode, and Coldplay, it's just that I felt my little contribution to these giant puzzles really didn't wake me up in the morning feeling inspired. I got up and did my duty every day, but I did so by default and with a cup of coffee from a local Starbucks where the barista knew my name and had my order ready upon seeing me.

There was something about being in Ram Dass's living room on that morning that really felt big to me. It felt beautiful. It felt complete. When Ram Dass woke up, I saw him like I had never seen him before. He appeared to me for the first time as my teacher. He knew! And he knew that I wanted to know! And that was enough of a hit for me to change the course for the rest of my life. I had spent so much time with him in my youth and early adulthood but never really resonated with his natural and seemingly unconditional spiritual love. I didn't know what my path would look like or exactly what it is I would do, but I did know that my current situation wasn't it. I later came to understand a great Ram Dass teaching that says the path of dharma is just as much about finding out what you don't want to do as much as it is what you do want to do.

Getting in touch with what really lights your fire and opens up your heart is a subtle and possibly long process. It's not one that will come to you overnight; it takes time. It takes a refinement of the skill of deeply listening to your intuition. If we sit still long enough and deeply listen to those little voices inside of our hearts that tell us what we should attract and what energy we should gently push away, things become a lot more harmonious.

The real life-changing moment of my trip to Maui wasn't just centered around my career. The trip opened me up to a whole new way of life. I became instantly immersed and in love with the path of bhakti yoga, a practice of devotion that I was first introduced to when I was sixteen years old. I knew who Neem Karoli Baba was thanks to reading *Be Here Now* and following the Grateful Dead around the country, but I never really had much interest in the guru system. This is probably because my parents had a great disdain for it. They did not like power structures or systems that seemed to strip away individuality and give power away to other people.

It's hard to know what was going on in Timothy's mind on a personal level, but nearly twenty-five years since he passed, my assumption is that he really misunderstood the guru system; he saw it as cultish and as a gimmick. When Ram Dass came back from India in 1968, I think Timothy certainly loved his friend but rolled his eyes at what he had become. I think if my father had a little bit of a softer heart and done more to heal his own personal pains, he would have had more openness and compassion for Eastern spiritual practices the same way he embraced the practice of psychedelic exploration.

The great irony for me personally is that I have the best of both worlds now. I have the deep intellectual seduction of philosophical materialism and the soft heart and unconditional love of bhakti yoga. I see no reason why the two can't live together in perfect harmony. It isn't a matter of choosing one over the other. Furthermore, when you really explore the Hindu Vedas and the idea of non-duality, you can see that the path of knowledge and the path of grace is really one and the same. The methods might look a little different, but the end goal gets us to the same place: a path that brings us to oneness with ourselves and in equanimity with the world around us.

For the next eleven years, my relationship with Ram Dass, primarily as a student but also as his friend, had an impact on me that words cannot express. It's almost as if I was given a chance to become a new me. I am not suggesting that those who find fulfillment in corporate life are fooling themselves and should quit their jobs to do whatever they want. I am saying that the quest for fulfillment is more important than that of accomplishment in the long term. And I hope my sudden 180 in my own life embodies that.

A few years later, I also found the confidence to embrace my roots and family lineage. The beauty of dancing around confused and lost early in life can have great rewards if you can manage to course-correct later on. I thank the gods that I was confused and lost, that I struggled with addiction, that I worked in Corporate America, that I pushed away everything that was being presented to me because I was fearful and felt I had no voice. Fortunately, I was able to sit still long enough to listen to what was being told to me in the quiet voice that is our intuition. The psychedelic world opened up to me once again, this time with a voice that had clarity and strong opinions—ones that sometimes were at polar opposites of my father's earlier work, which was entirely refreshing. This meant I could find a place in this world that was entirely my own. Influenced and even inspired by Timothy? Of course. But I am confident that I am not parroting his views or trying to copy his work.

All of these years later, having worked with countless psychedelic voyagers across the globe, hosted over three hundred podcast episodes, spoken at dozens of conferences on psychedelics, and had over two hundred personal psychedelic experiences, I feel pretty comfortable knowing where my passion lies and how I can contribute most effectively. Most important to me is not letting the mystical part of the psychedelic experience fall by the wayside as a new dawn of often sterilized medical psychedelic use emerges. While the mental health aspect of psychedelic use has become more and more effective, we must never lose sight of the fact that the use of psychedelic drugs is, in and of itself, mystical in nature. Policy issues around the legalization of psychedelics, ensuring proper and sound education around safe and effective use, changing the fear-based propaganda narratives that have seeped into public consciousness, and providing frameworks for compassionate, safe, and cautious use are also part of my mission.

I trust that all of this is reflected in the work that you are about to read.

1

The Language of the Medicine

A Glorious Mystery

"There's a space beyond language, it's just so damn hard to talk about."

—Terence McKenna

There have been a number of great books, documentaries, TED Talks, and endless podcasts that have detailed the rigorous recent scientific research that explains how psychedelic drugs work on the brain. In this golden age of psychedelic research, we have seen studies that have done fMRI scans of a brain under the influence of psilocybin and LSD, there are studies on how ketamine acts as a brain reset for those suffering with mental health issues, and very compelling studies exist that show us how and why the 5-HT2A receptor site in our brains that governs serotonin is remarkably similar to that of the psilocybin molecule. How someone sat for an fMRI brain scan while high on LSD is beyond me, but that's another story.

As conclusive, compelling, and wondrous as this new knowledge into how psychedelics work on the brain is, it still doesn't explain the unknown noetic induction into the mystical experience that opens up an entire world of possibilities when one is experiencing these medicines. And to make these mystical experiences even more elusive and illuminating, each of the major psychedelic drug categories speaks in its own style of unique language. The conversation you will have with yourself and spirit on LSD is far different than the one you'd have on MDMA or Ayahuasca. Each substance is a unique tapestry that requires getting to know its framework, sensibilities, and language. At first, taking it may feel like a roller coaster of lack of control, but when done right, it can morph beautifully into an endless stream of bliss, knowledge, and ancient wisdom and a view into the cosmic mirror that is your own consciousness.

Before we explore how these remarkable drugs can open up a window that allows you to have a conversation with long-forgotten parts of yourself or possibly with a source outside of your normal waking state, let's briefly explore what we know from a neuro-scientific perspective about how psychedelics work on the actual mechanisms of our brain.

As a matter of definitions and word choice, the words "entheogen" and "psychedelic" are used interchangeably throughout this book. Ralph Metzner, the great psychedelic researcher and Leary/Alpert partner at Harvard, says he prefers the word "entheogenic" because it's free from the cultural baggage that the word "psychedelic" has in our culture. Also, the word means "god within," and Metzner says it "refers explicitly to the capacity of these experiences to put one in touch with the sacred or divine dimensions of our existence."

The scientific research and effects on the brain shared in this book apply to entheogens like psilocybin, LSD, Ayahuasca, DMT, and mescaline. MDMA alters and then governs a similar portion of our brain but then does something that is unique unto itself and thus very different from a classic entheogen. As does ketamine, which is perhaps the most accessible new psychedelic agent because of its legal designation. Ketamine, it is worth pointing out, is not a true psychedelic by definition. It is an anesthetic dissociative that, when administered in lower doses, elicits psychedelic properties. It has been granted the label of a psychedelic purely by convenience, but that has shown to offer up a great amount of confusion around users who are new to this field.

For decades, researchers have been captivated by the profound effects that psychedelics can have on consciousness, but they had few tools available to understand how they worked on the brain until very recently. My own father, Timothy Leary, was so jolted by the possibilities that he left a senior post at Harvard University and the role of traditional psychologist to explore the issue. From mind-altering experiences to potential therapeutic benefits, these substances have sparked curiosity and fueled scientific exploration that researchers such as the prolific Robin Carhart-Harris and Dr. Roland Griffiths at Johns Hopkins have helped us understand.

This Is Your Brain on Drugs

Studies using brain imaging techniques, such as functional magnetic resonance imaging (fMRI) and positron emission tomography (PET), have revealed that psychedelics enhance neural connectivity. Brain regions that are usually segregated and operate independently start to communicate more extensively. This heightened connectivity can explain the increased complexity of thoughts, vivid imagery, and synesthetic experiences often associated with psychedelic trips. This is quite startling information in comparison to the now comically infamous 1980s TV commercial that showed an egg in a frying pan and said, "This is your brain on drugs."

When I first saw images of these brain scans, I was awestruck seeing the entire brain working together in harmony rather than the typical waking state of left brain-right brain activity.

Robin Carhart-Harris, who supervised these studies at the Imperial College London, said, "In many ways, the brain in the LSD state resembles the state our brains were in when we were infants: free and unconstrained. This also makes sense when we consider the hyper-emotional and imaginative nature of an infant's mind."

Carhart-Harris's studies that revealed the brain's activity under the influence of LSD and psilocybin confirmed everything I had always suspected but never had proof of. Those of you who have had high-dose LSD experiences might relate. In these states of altered consciousness, it's as if your brain breaks free from its rigid input/output functions and turns into a wide-angle lens that takes in as much information as possible. This temporary feeling of expansiveness feels as though it's infinite—that the sensation of being truly aware is a glimpse into a perfect reality where your brain functions at an optimal level.

Plant medicines, like psilocybin mushrooms, potentially weave in the adaptogenic (stress fighting and balancing properties) powers of the mycelium network to increase the possibility of the neurogenic effect going a step further by creating permanent new neuronal networks. Meaning, we can actually reprogram old ideas and behaviors into new ways of thinking that are permanent. This is known as neuroplasticity or synaptic rewiring. A fascinating aspect of psychedelic action on the brain is its potential to induce neuroplasticity—the brain's ability to reorganize and form new neural connections. Studies suggest that psychedelics can promote synaptic plasticity, allowing for novel connections and information flow between brain regions. This rewiring of neural circuits may underlie the long-lasting changes in perception, cognition, and mental health reported by some users.

Serotonin and Psychedelics

At the core of understanding how psychedelics affect the brain lies the neurotransmitter serotonin. Serotonin plays a crucial role in regulating mood, perception, and cognition. Psychedelics, such as lysergic acid diethylamide (LSD), psilocybin (found in magic mushrooms), and dimethyltryptamine (DMT), interact with serotonin receptors in the brain.

You might be familiar with serotonin because of the selective serotonin reuptake inhibitor (SSRI) class of psychiatric drugs, like Prozac and Zoloft. SSRIs are most commonly used by the medical establishment in the treatment of depressive disorders, anxiety disorders, and a myriad of other common psychological conditions. They work by regulating how much serotonin the receptor sites can take in, essentially treating the symptoms of mental health disorders but not offering a long-term, transformational benefit.

While I am not in opposition to Western psychiatric medications like SSRIs, as a rule, I have (like so many others) come to believe that they are overprescribed and aren't as effective as the rates of prescriptions lead us to believe. Still, many of those suffering from a mental health crisis can find relief from SSRIs if they find themselves peering over the cliff into the abyss. With the mental health crisis in the United States being the epidemic it is, I would hope that everyone involved—ranging from the American Psychiatric Association and the Department of Veterans Affairs to your neighborhood general psychologist—would be open to the possibility that other methods to treat mental health issues, like psychedelics, may be more effective. The rates of long-term efficacy for traditional mental health treatments are so low that the only way we can go is up.

Psychedelics primarily target then activate the serotonin (5-HT2A) receptors, which are predominantly located in the cerebral cortex—the outer layer of the brain that's responsible for higher-level thinking. When a psychedelic substance binds to these receptors, it triggers a cascade of events that lead to altered perception and consciousness.

It is worth noting that the psilocybin molecule is nearly identical to the serotonin molecule. This similarity might imply a cosmic aha moment: that many of the health answers we are looking for lie in nature and plants. So, perhaps we should listen, much like the Amazonian healers do when they say the plants are our "teachers."

While the serotonin 2A receptor is the primary target of psychedelics, other serotonin receptors and neurotransmitter systems are also influenced. The interplay between serotonin, dopamine, glutamate, and other neurotransmitters contributes to the complex effects of these substances. Understanding these interactions may aid in developing targeted therapeutic applications for conditions like depression, anxiety, and addiction in the same way we look at traditional psychiatric medications; however, psychedelics' impact on mental health and well-being is more holistic than psychiatric medicines today.

The Default Mode Network, the Critical Period, and How We Can Rewire

But what prevents us from achieving a reset or rewiring of our brain on our own? It certainly isn't impossible. The biohacking community has made popular many methods like cold plunges, supplements, and breathing techniques, which have shown tremendous results in the increase of human optimization. Psychedelic research, however, has blown the lid wide open on the possibility that we can rewire our brains' neuronal networks in ways never before imaginable.

But how does this happen? What inside of our brains makes for this possibility? Enter the default mode network.

The default mode network (DMN) is a network of brain regions that is active when an individual is at rest or engaged in internal thoughts. It is our nervous system's way of telling us what reality is and isn't when in a waking state. So when psychedelics modulate the activity of the DMN, leading to its temporary dissolution or reduced connectivity, it's as if an entire new operating system and relationship with our experience of reality are possible. This disruption may account for the ego-dissolving, transcendent states, and profound self-reflection experienced during psychedelic journeys. This alteration of the DMN can also occur when one actively engages in other forms of disruptive non-ordinary states of consciousness practices, like meditation or intense breathwork. These methods are also very effective, and I'm not here to proclaim that one is superior than another, but I will say that psychedelics offer an accelerated doorway into a state that disrupts the DMN and offers lasting change.

The Critical Period

Another window into lasting change via the use of psychedelics is the opening of "the critical period," which neuroscientists have long sought to understand. Critical periods often refer to specific developmental stages during which an organism (e.g., humans or mice) can learn new things depending on their sensitivity to stimuli and life experiences.

Critical periods have been demonstrated to perform such functions as helping birds learn to sing and helping humans learn a new language. When trying to put this into context, I'm reminded of how children can learn a new language or complicated piano lessons much faster than an adult can. Their critical periods are wide open and thus make their brains much more adaptable to neurolinguistic and neuro-functional learning.

Dr. Gül Dölen, associate professor of neuroscience at the Johns Hopkins University School of Medicine, led some studies with mice that have shown that psychedelic drugs are linked by their common ability to reopen such critical periods. The length of time the critical period is open fluctuates from two days to four weeks depending on the psychedelic given to the subject. Ketamine lasted forty-eight hours, while psilocybin lasted two weeks.

Dölen says, "There is a window of time when the mammalian brain is far more susceptible and open to learning from the environment. This window will close at some point, and then the brain becomes much less open to new learning."

The Psychedelic Experience

Before we move into the more esoteric parts of the psychedelic experience, it's useful to have a basic understanding of how psychedelics can alter our brain's mechanisms. Here, I aim to recap only the most basic elements of how psychedelics work on the brain because, as I mentioned previously, there are entire books and now thousands of peer-reviewed studies on this information.

What I find most useful about many of these studies is that they show how the medicines light up myriad connections in our brain to seemingly form one big brain operating at near full capacity. In our waking state, the different regions of our brain are activated depending on what kind of person we are and what is happening around us—for example, our right and left brain tendencies and how our amygdala is activated during a fear response. On psychedelics, those distinctions are temporarily cast aside in favor of the communication networks in your brain accelerating and entering a state that expands their relationship with consciousness.

But what the science doesn't explain is why the healing experiences of psychedelics come in the form of messages, downloads, realizations, and a newfound spiritual awareness that wasn't previously available in our normal, day-to-day, waking state of life.

Michael Pollan, whose book *How to Change Your Mind* became an international sensation and helped many people open up to the potential of psychedelics, previously wrote primarily about food and the agricultural ecosystem that produces what we eat. When he set forth on the path of writing a book on psychedelics, he was surprised at what he learned from immersing himself in the culture and experiencing the medicines for himself.

He told me, "When I first shifted from food to psychedelics, I thought of it as a right-angled turn—abrupt. But of course both subjects concern our health (physical and mental), and both subjects are about our relationship to other species in nature. In both cases, we're looking at plants (and fungi) that we think we're using but in fact are using us. Symbiosis is at the heart of these relationships, and these plants have succeeded in evolution by gratifying our various desires: for nutrition, for beauty, for consciousness change."

As reported by nearly everyone who has used these magical compounds, there is some sort of sensation that induces a conversation with one's subconscious and allows for new insights into our emotions, behaviors, traumas, and ideas. Pollan is a great example of someone who set out to investigate something specific and came out of it with that and a whole lot more.

Our belief systems and emotional responses become so deeply ingrained into our minds' perception of reality that it's hard for them to become altered. When psychedelics shift these parts of ourselves, it can feel as if a huge weight has been lifted off our hearts and minds. One so great that we often feel a renewed sense of purpose and inspiration to live a fuller and more healthy life. For some people, that conversation isn't with our own subconscious but with something outside of ourselves. Call it spirit or a teacher that lives within the plant's molecule if you take a shamanic perspective. The healers of the Shipibo tribe of Peru, for example, formed an entire culture based on the belief that the plants are teachers and that Grandmother Ayahuasca is a disembodied truth teller who will show you the brutal but beautifully honest predicament of your situation—one that's not always easy to see.

Terence McKenna, a luminary in the exploration of altered states, once described the psychedelic experience as a profound encounter with the transcendent, a gateway to the numinous realms that lie beyond our ordinary perception. In the spirit of his insights, let us embark on a voyage into the realm of psychedelia, where time dissolves, perceptions are heightened, and the universe reveals its infinite wonders.

Like the scientific method of understanding how psychedelics work on the brain, the experience itself can be loosely distilled down to four essential qualities: the dissolution of boundaries, visions (hallucinatory and otherwise), altered states of viewing consciousness, and emotional expansion.

Dissolution of Boundaries

Dissolution of boundaries is a way of saying that everything you know as reality will turn itself inside out to reveal a totally new set of boundaries, thought patterns, and ways of perceiving the world and your place in it. As the mind opens up to the influence of entheogenic and synthetic psychedelic substances, the boundaries that define our sense of self and the external world begin to blur. The familiar concepts of "I" and "other" lose their rigid distinctions, leading to a profound sense of interconnectedness while simultaneously leading to a sense of confusion at the realization of the rigidness that keeps us in its grip in our normal state of being. The ego, that omnipresent narrator of our lives, retreats to the background, allowing a deeper communion with the collective consciousness of humanity, nature, and the cosmos. The illusion of separateness dissolves, and a unifying thread weaves together all existence.

Hallucinatory Visions and Space-Time Dissolution

Within the realms of the psychedelic experience, the mind becomes an artist, painting vivid and awe-inspiring visions upon the canvas of perception. The ordinary world transforms into a kaleidoscope of colors, patterns, and geometric forms. Walls breathe, trees dance, and time unfolds in nonlinear and nonsequential patterns. Symbolic archetypes emerge from the depths of the subconscious, revealing the timeless mythic underpinnings of the human psyche. Time ceases to exist as you melt into a world of pure nothingness. These hallucinatory visions carry a sense of numinosity, leaving the traveler awestruck and humbled by the mysteries of existence.

Expanded States of Consciousness

Usually the word "altered" precedes the word "consciousness" when talking about psychedelics. Sure, that is true—your sense of consciousness is altered, but I prefer the concept of expansion. I subscribe to the idea that consciousness is a disembodied stream of information, love, wisdom, and data that permeates every sentient being, and that our minds allow us to tap into that stream, thus giving us a sense of awareness—the "being aware that we are aware" sensation that pervades the human experience.

The psychedelic experience catapults the mind into expanded states of consciousness, where the boundaries of normal waking awareness are transcended and you can "see" a much greater sense of what is surrounding you at all times. Time becomes elastic, stretching and compressing, ultimately dissolving into an eternal present. Perception is amplified, unveiling hidden layers of reality that lie beyond the veil of our everyday senses. Profound insights and revelations flow into consciousness, shedding light on the nature of self, society, and the cosmos. The mind, liberated from its usual constraints, explores the vast, uncharted territories of existence.

Emotional Resonance

Within the psychedelic experience, emotions reverberate with heightened intensity. Joy, awe, love, and ecstasy can swell to unimaginable heights, enveloping the individual in a sea of euphoria. Simultaneously, the depths of sorrow, fear, and existential angst may also be plumbed, leading to transformative confrontations with one's inner demons. Emotions become a gateway to self-understanding and empathic connection, fostering compassion and empathy toward oneself and others. The full spectrum of human emotion unfolds, inviting profound catharsis and emotional integration.

The Power of Psychedelic Experiences

The psychedelic experience is a profound journey into the depths of consciousness, where the veils of ordinary perception are lifted, and the mysteries of existence are unveiled. It is an invitation to explore the interconnectedness of all things, to witness the splendor of hallucinatory visions, and to embrace the boundless realms of altered states. We can approach this transformative odyssey with reverence, curiosity, and an open heart, for it is through the psychedelic experience that we may touch the ineffable and discover the infinite tapestry of consciousness that unites us all.

From a scientific perspective, we have more questions than answers about how psychedelics work on an esoteric level. We have no hard data for why they produce the experiences they do and why the effects of these compounds leave us with a sense of transformation and insight into our own unique views of our humanity. It's worth considering that Indigenous cultures that used these plant medicines didn't ask why; they just gave way to the notion that the plants are teachers. By stopping to commune and listen to them, you can gain access to the vast mysteries of the universe.

The language of the medicine speaks in a voice that may sound like your own, but in truth it is a voice that is beyond language and beyond measurement. The more we try to study these medicines' effects on human consciousness, the more we realize that we will never truly grasp the wonders of how they alter our relationship with our own minds, emotions, nervous systems, and spiritual well-being. The "why" becomes less and less important when we listen to the experiences of others who have embarked on these transformational journeys.

Jason (names and identifying details have been changed throughout the book to protect privacy), a veteran I worked with who went through MDMA therapy to treat his PTSD, came to me to go even deeper by using psilocybin to help shed light on some unanswered questions. He recalled the following, "MDMA showed me that the actions that caused my PTSD weren't my fault but didn't do much to fill the spiritual hole left in my soul. I asked my facilitator to make sure to give me autobiographical cues during my session so I could make sense of them in some other way. What I got out of it went far beyond my past and those horrors—the medicine gave me a mantra-like affirmation that I am good, worthy, and part of a bigger something, a bigger something that I can't define, and I don't even like the word God. I feel like I met God for the first time. The messages were clear. MDMA eased the pain, but psilocybin brought me closer to stuff I didn't even know I was looking for."

In the realms of altered perception and expanded consciousness, the psychedelic experience stands as a remarkable doorway to the mysteries of the human mind. Like a shamanic journey into the depths of the psyche, it unveils a tapestry of visions, emotions, and insights. And in Jason's case, it brought a man in pain closer to a universal truth of interconnectedness in all beings and most importantly within himself.

In my own early experiences as a psychonaut, I was struck by these medicines' ability to pull back the curtain to reveal an entire other dimension of reality that can't be seen under normal conditions. And when I turned the lens on myself, it was as if I was being guided by some other voice that needed to show me what I was made of. It's very possible that voice may have been my own intuition and had nothing to do with spirit, or the complete opposite may be true. I still have no idea. But what I do know is that those formative years of exploration set the tone for a lifelong curriculum in the study of the place where my mind, heart, and spirit meet and talk in a language that far exceeds the predictability of English.

I'm also very grateful that I learned, even thirty-five years ago, that psychedelics aren't sustainable as a regular ritual of self-inquiry due to the fact that you must come down. But when used wisely, the sneak peek into this wisdom can be sustained through culture, personal practices, art, and community. The trip fades, but the transformation doesn't have to.

This ongoing process of transformation is what we now commonly refer to as "integration," which is the assigning of meaning to your psychedelic experience. We'll explore integration more fully later in the book, but it's what I like to describe as "sustainability"—the third "S" in the expansion of the paradigm we know as set and setting. Set, setting, and sustainability.

Exploring the subtle "language of the medicine" is important if you're curious about these drugs' effect on mental health because their efficacy lies in a complete 180 from the traditional approach. As mentioned earlier, the most common psychiatric Western medicines, like SSRIs (Prozac, Zoloft, etc.) and monoamine oxidase inhibitors (MAOIs, such as Nardil, Marplan, etc.) work by treating the symptoms of a disorder by altering a part of the brain through a pharmacological effect. Psychedelics do not create effective experiences by a chemical alteration alone, but also through deeper processes.

Of course the chemical in the drug does affect the brain, but the resulting experience goes far beyond a scientific explanation. The surreal, weird, otherworldly, and multidimensional ego/self varieties of the psychedelic state can't be scientifically explained no matter how hard we try.

In addition to understanding how psychedelics work on individuals, it's essential that we learn to decipher the language of the medicine in an interpersonal way. Everyone has their own relationship with the medicine journey that is theirs alone. Support and guidance from a skilled guide or facilitator can help make the use of psychedelics vital and long-lasting. This lack of skilled facilitation and integration contributed to the downfall of the 1960s psychedelic revolution. Millions of people got taken to the edge of the ecstatic cliff of expanded consciousness but were given no road map for how to get down. Sadly, most let their experiences die down and turned to the self-centered indulgence of the late '70s and '80s, as if their explorations were just novel recreations of the counterculture rather than profoundly transformative experiences.

But what are these "downloads" that we hear so much about? And what is it about these medicines that allow them to happen?

In a Johns Hopkins study of psilocybin for treatment-resistant depression, one of the participants, who goes by the name Vanessa, said of his experience, "I did not experience a peak experience or what they call an ego death," but he learned to identify the "self-limiting belief systems that have dominated his life" and "experienced spontaneous emotions that were not typical" for him.

This case is a valuable resource for those who are newer to these medicines and those who consider themselves to be atheists. Vanessa tones down the fantastical unity experience or one-with-God quality that others claim to have experienced in favor of talking about the pragmatic. Vanessa describes the benefits from his psilocybin treatments as useful and grounded realizations, yet he can't explain how or why the voices in his head took on the shape and color that they did. He is pinpointed and specific about how useful the psilocybin treatments were in combating his lifelong depression and expressed it in a way that is accessible for everyone, whether they're on a spiritual path or not.

Learning how to let the medicine speak to you in a way that is unique unto yourself is perhaps the greatest experiential technique to cultivate to have healing psychedelic journeys. And if there's any one technique that I wish I could teach others, it would be this. But it has to be learned by yourself. Guides, therapists, shamans, and mystics can give you a framework for best practices, but they can't tell you any one way to do it.

2

Psychedelic Substances

How They Can Change
Your World Inside and Out

"Psychedelics, used responsibly and with proper caution,
would be for psychiatry what the microscope is for biology
and medicine or the telescope is for astronomy."

—Stanislav Grof

The plant medicines like psilocybin mushrooms, Ayahuasca, and peyote have been used for so long that they are practically woven into the DNA of human evolution. As I'll discuss in more detail later, somewhere down the line, most of us have an ancestral relative that used these medicines as part ritual and part medicine. They are just as much part of the human story as tracing our relationship to food and agriculture.

The newer synthetic compounds like LSD and MDMA don't have centuries of tribal connection; therefore, their histories and impact on our evolution isn't as pronounced. But on the flip side, our history with these drugs is still being written in real time. They aren't part of the natural world, but now and then humankind gets it right and stumbles into an invention, a molecule, or a theory that changes the very course of evolution. Such as it is with LSD and MDMA. These drugs are spirit molecules that are the result of humankind's quest to search for meaning in its various manifestations.

Getting to Know Each Substance

Each of the major compounds I talk about in this chapter has its own language. Each pierces the veil of human consciousness to expand our relationship with our surroundings and ourselves, but they do so in unique ways. Each may change you in ways that are similar in the long run, but the path to get there is wildly different. I like to say that each of the main psychedelic drugs are like different rides in the same amusement park. It's A Small World is a very different experience than Space Mountain, but both are at Disneyland and both usher in that certain brand of Disney's make-believe formula. A loose metaphor for sure, but you get the point.

In this chapter, it seems only appropriate and authentic that I cover the psychedelic drugs that I have the most experience with on a deeply personal level. Each one of these compounds has changed me and helped make me the person I am today. As we discuss the elements of the drugs and their psychoactive effects, I feel it's important to also include why one should consider taking them in the first place. The history, cultural impact, legal melodramas, and personal intention are all parts of the story for each drug. In this chapter, I will break down the following aspects of each drug: its cultural roots, reasons for taking it, possible contraindications, and suggested ways in which you can make the most out of taking it. Each drug discussed is followed by a series of questions. Answering these questions with sincerity will get you closer to creating a symbiotic relationship with the drug should you choose to use it.

The disclaimer on the bottle for any of these substances would read: "Before any psychedelic drug is to be considered for personal and/or therapeutic use, your most impactful intentions around taking them must be verbalized and expressed with great clarity. If you do not know why you want to take these drugs, then you should not be taking them." What can they offer you that you could not otherwise find elsewhere? After those intentions are isolated, it's vital to maintain objectivity around both the positive and cautionary aspects of using these drugs.

With that in mind, it is also necessary to point out that not all psychedelics are right for all people. Getting clear on that takes a tremendous amount of research and honest insight into your own individual calibration. For instance, if you have never taken MDMA, do some research on it, talk to people who have taken it, understand its pros and cons, and then if you feel like it is not the right fit for you, by all means do not take it. And if you've done all that and feel like it is a promising option for your healing or growth, then make sure you understand the correct usage protocols and make sure you trust the procurement source to ensure drug purity. Impure drugs have set the movement back time and time again. DanceSafe is an easy-to-use website that sells at-home testing kits for a variety of psychedelic drugs. They operate from a harm-reduction standpoint, and I can't recommend using their products enough.

LSD

When writing about synthetic compounds like LSD or MDMA, a realization of deep emotional significance washed over me like a tidal wave. Plant medicine aficionados will be quick to point out that compounds like psilocybin and Ayahuasca have been woven into the human story for thousands of years, and because of that, their use has been tested for countless generations. Synthetic compounds do not have that connection. They are new and thus do not share intergenerational connections with us. However, when I look within and take note of how God works, I am left with the realization that God speaks through our minds, our art, and our inventions. LSD is a spirit molecule that was left for us to discover in order to spark our evolutionary potential. Just because it is new that does not mean it has to be thought of as any less ceremonial. We are the ones who will set the tone for how generations to come can use the medicine of LSD and other synthetic compounds. We must remember that and use them with the same reverence as the ancient plant medicine cultures have taught us.

Out of all the substances, LSD is nearly impossible for me to look at objectively due to the ironclad grip of its historical claws that caused my family great persecution. I wouldn't be where I am today if it weren't for LSD. It changed me personally in ways that I can't begin to describe (but I'll try) and helped pave a path forward for people like me to actually have a career in psychedelics.

Swiss chemist Albert Hofmann's synthesis of LSD at Sandoz Laboratories in 1938 made apparent the limitless potential of the drug's psychotherapeutic value, thanks to Hofmann's own ingestion of the molecule in April 1943. But it was so volatile that Hofmann himself called it "my problem child." Hearing that always reminds me of Oppenheimer's now infamous quoting of the Bhagavad Gita after watching the first atomic bomb test: "I am become death, the destroyer of worlds." Sometimes human beings stumble into something so vast and limitless in application that the effects that follow leave us with wondrous panic and a healthy fear of the well-intentioned invention.

Because of the powerful psychological shift LSD had the potential to create, control of the drug in the US fell into the hands of various government agencies that ushered in stranger-than-fiction CIA-sponsored programs like MK-ULTRA—a black ops mission that was tasked with creating new mind-control programs that could be used on the battlefield to go inside enemies' minds and get information rather than flat out killing them. Once again, LSD proved to be unpredictable for those uses and seemed to make the test subjects laugh and howl more than it made them scream and recoil in terror.

Fortunately, on a parallel path, LSD's still-legal status in the 1950s meant that the therapeutic value was being tested (quite successfully) by early clinical psychology mavericks like Dr. Oz Janiger and Dr. Humphry Osmond. The documentary *Becoming Cary Grant*, which is a starkly vulnerable autobiographical romp through the life of film icon Cary Grant, portrayed the use of LSD in a clinical setting in the 1950s. It made fine work of documenting the early successes of LSD in an intentional, transformational, and therapeutic setting.

Working with the Beverly Hills–based doctor Mortimer Hartman, who was administering LSD to his patients, Grant recounted in his own words how LSD became the mirror in which he could view his own life and identity issues. "After weeks of treatment came a day when I saw the light," he said in the film. "When I broke through, I felt an immeasurably beneficial cleansing of so many needless fears and guilts. I lost all the tension that I'd been crippling myself with. First I thought of all those wasted years. Second, I said, 'Oh my God, the humanity. Please come in.'"

LSD is also the drug that blew the psychedelic movement wide open and brought it to the mainstream. People like Rick Doblin, the founder of MAPS, said that in the '60s "psychedelic drugs leaked from the laboratory and with that came misuse." There is some truth to that statement, but the pros far outweigh the cons.

As discussed earlier, prior to youth culture's adoption of drugs like LSD and cannabis in the 1960s, 1950s America was an alcohol- and nicotine-driven society that made no room for other intoxicants. Those other intoxicants were demonized, misunderstood, and when used, pierced the veil into the conformist absurdity of post-war America and its white picket fence dream. But when Leary, Alpert, Kesey, and the rest shouted from the mountaintop that LSD was the most powerful tool ever discovered to study the human mind and consciousness, the divide became so deep that an immediate us-versus-them paradigm began, which contributed to the anti-Vietnam war movement and the modern DEA (Drug Enforcement Administration). The old guard saw these drugs as a threat and rightly so. Suddenly, millions of young people were questioning authority and rejecting the old ways of being told how to live their life. They weren't going to be forced to fight an unwinnable foreign war or keep quiet while Black Americans were persecuted merely for being Black. The culture wars had begun!

My father, Timothy Leary, was heralded as the acid king of the '60s and was both praised and vilified for his role in the drug's proliferation. One side viewed him as one of the great thinkers of the twentieth century—as a man who encouraged a generation to think for themselves and question authority by looking at the way the mind operates. And on the other hand, President Nixon called him the "most dangerous man in America." Where the truth lies is up to the observer. I'm not here to comment on that. However, his role in making LSD what it is today is essential in understanding the history of LSD. Synonymous with the Grateful Dead, The Beatles, and the entire counterculture movement, LSD has been linked with everything from the inspiring message of *Sgt. Pepper's* to urban legends of people believing they had grown wings and could jump off a building. There is a lot of room between those two things.

The only ancient lineage of LSD is fuzzy, stemming from folklorish tales of rye rotting and forming a mysterious substance. Ergot of rye fungus contains traits of the same compound as lysergic acid diethylamide but offers up a host of other less-appealing reactions, like convulsions. But still, tales from the Salem witch trials of 1692 have their roots in a mysterious fungus that was contaminating the town's rye bread supply causing "ergotism." Did that fungus, a relative of LSD, cause the townsfolk to have visions of witchcraft? Quite possibly, yes! The village doctor, being religious and thus a believer in evil supernatural powers, unaware of ergotism, attributed the women's symptoms to what he saw as a known evil: witchcraft. It wasn't until Swiss chemist Albert Hofmann synthesized the drug for Sandoz Labs in 1938 did the purposeful use of LSD begin to form a road map. Even that didn't happen right away. Hofmann's now famous bicycle ride of 1943—in which he rode his bicycle home from the lab after accidentally ingesting his creation—was the first time the psychedelic effects of the drug were felt and thus began a beautiful chemical love story that has altered the lives of millions of people around the globe.

It's a funny thing that a chemical compound engineered in the twentieth century can produce experiences of divinity that bring up ancient messages that transcend generations. It begs the question: Where does divinity lie? Is it hidden deep within the wells of human innovation, begging for us to figure out how to unlock it? It's almost as if God Herself is playing a fun little game by hiding the keys to the kingdom and making us play hide-and-seek. One of the ways we must figure out where the keys are hidden is by using our ingenuity to invent a mechanism that finds the key and then makes it usable. What a mindfuck! Nonetheless, it is true. Anyone who has used LSD with positive results will claim that they understood themselves and the universe around them much more holistically than they had prior to taking the drug. The feeling of "All One" is often experienced after a good LSD trip—a sensation of feeling your uniqueness but also your place in the collective cosmic order of things.

Because of the wide variety of possible experiences the LSD spectrum has to offer, pinpointing intent is essential. When I was in my teens, my friends and I would go to "Yes Land"—a place that required 250 micrograms of good LSD, a tank full of nitrous oxide, and a CD carousel full of music by the progressive rock band YES. Our intent was to commune with the outer realms of the collective conscious and dance among the stars. Just a few years later, with the same dosage but without the music, my intention was to confront my inner demons head on so I could best make sense of why I do the things I do. When altering the "set and setting" only slightly, the experience influences intent and vice versa. Bottom line, LSD is a confrontational drug, not an escapist one. External surroundings play an important role in determining what you'll get in the end.

The deepest work I've done on LSD has shown me parts of myself that I find almost hard to talk about. Why, when in active addiction, do I turn into a person I don't want to be and cause harm to others? Those eight hours on the drug epitomize the dark night of the soul and your willingness to change. After coming down, I've found it essential to not deny those dark realizations and to instead write them down and be up front with my humanity, even if it's painful. When writing down rigorously honest road maps before and after LSD journeys, I've seen (with myself and the clients I work with) that intention is the only way to stop yourself from coming down and forgetting that any of it happened.

I recommend substantial doses of LSD only for strong and stable personalities. Those suffering from mental health issues or those who lack a sense of self-worth and purpose can easily be thrown into the hand of the lysergic demon. Radical self-love, stability in internal and external areas of one's life, and a strong spiritual connection are absolute essentials in defining a quality "set and setting" for an LSD trip. If anyone lacks any of those elements, I encourage them to be cautious and wait to take an LSD trip.

Pre-LSD Journey Questions to Ask Yourself

1. Is the drug pure? Do you trust the source? Have you tested it? (Testing kits are available at dancesafe.com.)

2. Is the dosage for the LSD you've obtained labeled? (Remember, we are dealing with micrograms, so the dosage matters!)

3. Why do you want to use LSD in the first place? Are you clear about your intentions?

4. Describe any fears that you have around taking LSD (both mental and physical).

5. What's your plan for taking it? What dosage? When, where, and with a guide or with friends? If working with a guide, are they well trusted and with a good reputation?

6. Are you in good health and feel that you can withstand the intensity of LSD? If not, be honest about it and recognize that this medicine might not be right for you.

7. What is your integration plan? What are you going to do in the hours and days afterward?

MDMA

> "MDMA gives you a new perspective on yourself.
> It lets you see that love, even self-love, is
> something you can experience."

—Ann Shulgin

MDMA has become synonymous within the counterculture as the "feel good" drug or "the love drug." In fact, Timothy Leary once stated that two people who do MDMA together should not get married until a forty-eight-hour window has passed.

The now legendary psychopharmacologist Alexander "Sasha" Shulgin is credited with synthesizing MDMA in the late '60s and refining its disinhibiting effects in the '70s. He saw it as a powerful aid in therapy. He did not invent the drug, however. Its roots go back to the pharma giant Merck in 1912, with a reemergence by the US Army in the 1950s. I find it a powerful footnote that many of our chemical psychedelic friends, including MDMA and LSD, have their roots in the military and Big Pharma. Don't forget, Albert Hofmann was working for Sandoz at the time of his famous bicycle ride.

MDMA allows the receptor sites in your brain to increase the flow of serotonin and dopamine in such a radical way that it (temporarily) allows the user to reassociate trauma centers away from pain and toward measurable social rewards. This is why MDMA is so effective in treating PTSD: the user can literally experience a heart-opening and empathetic flood of love that allows them to see the cause of their PTSD in a whole new way.

Mapping out your intentions when taking MDMA can be especially helpful because it is essential to understand that the experience on the drug, the trip itself, is very temporary. The high has very precise peaks and comedowns. If you don't map out your intention beforehand then follow it up with writing afterward, you run the risk of getting hung up on that ultra-euphoric high that you experienced for a mere three to five hours that then dissipates. Again, the real work begins after the session. The session itself is just the liftoff that will expose you to new and better conditions.

So, what draws you to MDMA? Let's look at a range of intentions that are based on "vibrational payoff" points—that is, from low vibe to high vibe. There is nothing inherently wrong with pursuing low-vibe pleasure, but one must be aware that the long-term, cost-benefit payoff will remain low, even fleeting. On the other hand, the risk-to-reward ratio will be much higher, even life-changing, if you are using MDMA for a highly vibrational reason. Real-life scenarios might include taking MDMA at a rave (low vibe) to using MDMA to heal past traumas (high vibe). There are lots of places in between those two examples, which is what's great about the psychedelic experience. It can be custom-tailored to suit your personal set of circumstances.

Taking MDMA tends to cause euphoria, increased empathy to oneself and others, lack of judgment, physical pleasure, heart-centeredness, auditory bliss, and visual flutters. The pros of the MDMA experience are often the ability to love more, intense euphoria, and the ability to develop a new relationship with past traumas. Cons for some users can include a post-session hangover, mild depression, tendency for overuse, and neurotoxicity. Neuroscientific studies have shown that MDMA is taxing on the brain's serotonin axons; however, the degree of neurotoxicity is inconclusive. Countless peer-reviewed studies on both humans and animals suggest the same thing: MDMA abuse is not a good idea, while moderate and safe MDMA use will not permanently harm the user.

There are fewer studies on how to prevent unwanted side effects from taking MDMA, but research and experience suggests that taking certain precautions can reduce your post-session drawbacks. Supplements like 5-HTP and L-tryptophan, when combined with a converting catalyst like vitamin B6, are effective ways to prep the serotonin axon blocks from depletion before a session and replenish the same blocks after a trip quicker than without the supplements, thus reducing the depression that may be experienced after a trip.

These supplements can be found on their own; however, the bio-hacking company founded by Aubrey Marcus, Onnit, makes a product called "New Mood" that contains all of these and more. Taking two pills a day for two days prior to an MDMA session (but stopping the day before) and two pills a day for three days after will make the session much smoother and reduce the amount of "burn" you feel after. I recommend, if not insist, that well-intentioned MDMA users follow a similar protocol to ensure the safest and most productive results. There are many MDMA usage protocols out there; this is one I recommend. I encourage you to further your research before embarking on the use of this drug.

Pre-MDMA Journey Questions to Ask Yourself

1. Is the drug pure? Do you trust the source? Have you tested it? (Testing kits are available at dancesafe.com.)

2. Are you planning to engage in the pre- and post-session supplement protocol recommended for MDMA use? If not, why?

3. Why do you want to use MDMA in the first place? Are you clear about your intentions? Do you feel that taking MDMA is in alignment with realizing your highest sense of self?

4. Do you feel that you are an empathetic person to begin with? Are you in touch with your heart space as it relates to yourself and other people in your life?

5. Knowing that MDMA will expand your heart space, what do you want to get from that experience?

6. If you are using MDMA to heal trauma, describe the trauma. Don't hold back, keep it real.

7. What's your plan for taking it? What dosage? When, where, and with a guide or with friends? If working with a guide, are they well trusted and with a good reputation?

8. Describe any fears, mental or physical, that you have around taking MDMA.

9. Are you in good health and feel that you can withstand the intensity of MDMA? If not, be honest about it and recognize that this medicine might not be right for you.

10. What is your integration plan? What are you going to do in the hours and days afterward?

Psilocybin

Psychedelic mushrooms, such as *Psilocybe cubensis*, are perhaps the most widely used and globally proliferated plant medicine for sacramental uses—not only among ancient cultures but also today. From Maya and Mexica all the way to Siberia, hallucinogenic mushrooms have had a range of uses, from preserving oral traditions, bonding with tribal communities, and having a direct experience with God to staying warm in inhospitable climates. There's even evidence that suggests ancient Romans during their pagan heyday had an appetite for psychedelic mushrooms.

Because of the ancient lineage of these sacraments, the idea of intention has evolved to meet the times that the individual finds themselves in. The idea of taking mushrooms today in order to get in touch with our ancestral elders so they might whisper ancient wisdom into our subconscious is in a way de-evolution. It's a return to a human way of being that hasn't existed for millennia. This is a radical concept. Our brains, stimuli, and relationship dynamics would be almost unrecognizable to our ancestors. Taking the same psychedelic plant that they took might help us experience a simpler way of life that emphasizes a focus on love, our environment, community, and respect. A little de-evolution is not a bad thing in this context. Humans today take in more stimulus per second than at any time in history, and who knows how this will impact our future selves. The marvels of the modern world are mystical wonders in and of themselves, but when we are given the opportunity to reset our relationship with them, these wonders of innovation take on a different purpose.

To me, revisiting ancient wisdom and concepts of enlightenment and fusing that with our place in the modern world is the heart of intent in the current application of psilocybin use. Psilocybin can help us get in touch with an idea of divinity that is pure, a concept of the divine that will help us heal from the traumas of the modern world—whether external or interpersonal.

When taking psilocybin, it's important to pay attention to both the variety and species of mushroom as well as the dosage. Twenty years ago, it wasn't as easy to have so many varieties of psilocybin mushrooms to choose from, and they were more or less consistent in terms of potency. For example, one gram was a very moderate social dose, two grams was a deeper but non-ego-dissolving dose, and four-to-five grams and up was a heroic dose that may induce ego dissolution and required much more attention to setting.

Today, it's not quite that simple. For instance, two grams of Penis Envy psilocybin mushrooms is not the same as two grams of Golden Teachers. Penis Envy mushrooms are a variety within the *Psilocybe cubensis* (*p. cubensis*) family of shrooms. But this is no ordinary *Psilocybe cubensis* mushroom; it's exceptionally potent. The psilocin and psilocybin content (what makes these mushrooms psychoactive) can be as high as 2.9 percent. In comparison, Golden Teachers produce between 0.5 and 0.9 percent.

The difference in potency is huge and cannot be ignored, so please make sure you know what strain you are dealing with before plotting your dosage. There are many online guides for different strains of mushrooms; Double Blind, Third Wave, and Shroomer are all good places to start.

Pre-Psilocybin Journey Questions to Ask Yourself

1. What strain of mushroom have you obtained? Are you familiar with its potency? Remember all strains do not contain the same level of psilocin and psilocybin.

2. Why do you want to use psilocybin in the first place? Are you clear about your intentions? Do you feel that taking psilocybin is in alignment with realizing your highest sense of self?

3. Do you have a working knowledge of and respect for the Indigenous use of psilocybin mushrooms?

4. If you are using psilocybin for mental health reasons, have you educated yourself on the most current clinical trials and their outcomes (i.e., Johns Hopkins, NYU, etc.)?

5. What's your plan for taking it? What dosage? When, where, and with a guide or with friends? If working with a guide, are they well trusted and with a good reputation?

6. Describe any fears, mental or physical, that you have around taking psilocybin.

7. Are you in good health and feel that you can withstand the intensity of psilocybin? If not, be honest about it and recognize that this medicine might not be right for you.

8. What is your integration plan? What are you going to do in the hours and days afterward?

DMT/5-MeO-DMT

"I think that drugs should be as noninvasive as possible, and I know I'm on the right track because the strongest psychedelic drugs are the ones that last the shortest amount of time. Now, what does that mean? It means that your brain recognizes the compound and within a few minutes can completely neutralize it. DMT is the strongest psychedelic there is, yet it lasts only five minutes. Twenty minutes after you do it, it's like you never did it at all."

—Terence McKenna

The dimethyltryptamine (DMT) molecule, of all the psychedelic compounds, is both the most powerful and the shortest acting. Because of those two factors, there sometimes is an attraction to doing it often. On the other hand, with the 5-MeO version of DMT, the experience can be so insanely disorienting and wildly psychedelic that a complete ego death occurs, and the user might come back and never want to get near it again. It was simply too much.

Too much of what, though?

The only way I can describe DMT's effects is an express ticket to pure consciousness. A place where the veil between waking reality and cosmic awareness gets lifted so quickly that you are shot on a rocket ship to a world that is full of gorgeous sacred geometry, complete loss of awareness surrounding your physical body, and a place where your thinking mind ceases to exist and turns into a vehicle of awareness.

Words really do it no justice.

Some say it is a doorway to an ancient language left to us from alien ancestors, while others say it is a speedway to the face of the divine. Mystical experiences, spiritual ones, alien contact, or pure ego death—it's hard to say. Somewhere in between all of these lies the truth because from an experiential standpoint, the results are purely subjective.

DMT has roots in ancient cultures as a ritual psychedelic, making it an entheogen. It is usually smoked, so the high comes on very quickly and doesn't last long. Contemporary users have called it the "businessman's LSD" because of these traits. However, the Indigenous cultural roots of DMT are more complex. The molecule that makes DMT can be found in Amazonian plants that natives used in ceremonies.

DMT as we know it now was first synthesized in 1931 by chemist Richard Helmuth Frederick Manske, but the psychedelic/hallucinogenic properties weren't isolated until 1956 by Hungarian chemist Stephen Szára. Rick Strassman, author of *DMT: The Spirit Molecule* stated: "My studies with DMT and psilocybin were not therapeutic. Nevertheless, I had spiritual questions and an orientation that was brought to our studies. I came from a spiritual perspective developed over twenty years of Zen study and practice. Therefore, I expected mystical-unitive experiences as a result of a high dose of DMT. However, only one out of nearly five dozen volunteers had what might be considered this type of effect—and he was a religious studies major in college who had always wished for a mystical state. A mystical-unitive state did not occur in any other volunteer, so one might not consider its effects to be spiritual at all. Contrary to the mystical state, our volunteers interacted with a highly articulated 'world' that often felt 'inhabited' and 'more real' than consensus reality."

Strassman's extensive research with DMT is one of the only legal studies to be granted, and as you can see by his statement, the effects of the drug are purely subjective. Some may claim to see the face of God, while others see a constructed reality that, while describable, is completely different from our normal one.

Terence McKenna stated in *The Archaic Revival,* "DMT was so much more powerful, so much more alien, raising all kinds of issues about what is reality, what is language, what is the self, what is three-dimensional space and time, all the questions I became involved with over the next twenty years or so."

Because it can be challenging to explain what the experience of DMT is like, and because people have such a wide variety of experiences, DMT can be challenging to recommend for healing purposes. That doesn't mean it shouldn't be used therapeutically; it's just harder to explain why it should be. Many veterans, for instance, have used 5-MeO-DMT at healing centers designed to treat vets specifically, and most come back saying they felt "lighter" and went through an experience that purged them of some of the somatic residue that their

PTSD held. There can be tremendous spiritual value in visiting the "spirit molecule." Being jettisoned out of the normal confines of waking reality to bring you closer to God, alien beings, sacred geometry, or other psychedelic worlds has benefits because it gives you the opportunity to pierce the veil and see what's underneath. That is no small matter.

In *The Archaic Revival*, McKenna went on to say, "The reason it's so confounding is because its impact is on the language-forming capacity itself. So the reason it's so confounding is because the thing that is trying to look at the DMT is infected by it—by the process of inspection. So DMT does not provide an experience that you analyze. Nothing so tidy goes on. The syntactical machinery of description undergoes some sort of hyper-dimensional inflation instantly, and then, you know, you cannot tell yourself what it is that you understand. In other words, what DMT does can't be downloaded into as low-dimensional a language as English."

From what I can tell and with everything I've researched, our grip on our perceived reality creates an attachment paradigm that is so firm that any alteration of it makes us think we are "losing one's grip." I think there is an enormous benefit to being shown the other side, to losing one's grip, in a very controlled, short-acting setting. It can give relief and a sense of satisfaction to see that nothing is what it seems. This, in turn, can grant us a long-term relationship with joy, love, a sense of oneness, and an overall green light to not take everything so seriously. Once you see that the universe is all controlled chaos, suddenly the anxiety around paying your phone bill late doesn't hold much water.

Defining intention for something that is so amorphous in description and elastic in reality makes any planning to take DMT difficult. But not impossible. The following questions, I believe, will help you unpack your desire to be an explorer of the outer limbs of the self-contained universe (or multiverse). Mapping out a plan ahead of time—in writing, the best you can—will hopefully make the "beyond language" trip itself have some kind of meaning and therefore provide growth.

Pre-DMT Journey Questions to Ask Yourself

1. Is the drug pure? Do you trust the source?

2. Why do you want to use DMT in the first place? Are you clear about your intentions? Do you feel that taking DMT is in alignment with realizing your highest sense of self?

3. Are you positive that you know what you're getting into? Remember, this is the most powerful psychedelic known to man. Your ego will disappear for anywhere from ten to twenty minutes.

4. What's your plan for taking it? When, where, and how much?

5. What is your method of intake? Smoking? Vaping? Each one delivers a different potency.

6. Who is going to sit for you while you take the drug? You should *never* do this drug alone.

7. Describe any fears, mental or physical, that you have around taking DMT.

8. Are you in good health and feel that you can withstand the intensity of DMT? If not, be honest about it and recognize that this medicine might not be right for you.

9. What is your integration plan? What are you going to do in the hours and days afterward?

Ayahuasca

I am not an initiate of any Ayahuasca lineage, such as the Shipibo tribe of Peru or the Santo Daime Church of Brazil. My knowledge of Ayahuasca is limited to two personal experiences and a fair amount of academic knowledge. I do not consider myself to be an expert on this amazing plant medicine in any shape or form. Because of that, the pre-journey questions that I provide are more generalized to fit any psychedelic experience that you are about to go on. The in-depth process of going on an Ayahuasca journey is better left to the healers and Indigenous tribes that are keeping the integrity of Ayahuasca use alive and well.

There is only one suggestion that I have when considering if Ayahuasca is right for you: do it under the supervision and guidance of a healer that has been initiated into any one of the many Ayahuasca lineages. This does not mean a self-styled, new age guru who calls themselves a shaman or priest or priestess. Specifically, only trust a healer who has long and legitimate connections to an Indigenous tribe of South America. Also, please do your research on who this person is and the integrity of their offering at any one of the many Ayahuasca retreat centers. There have been tales of abuse on many levels, and committing to the process of an entire Ayahuasca ceremony is a deeply intimate and vulnerable thing to do. Choose wisely.

I say this because there is a growing number of Westerners who have become so deeply moved and impassioned from their Ayahuasca use that they have taken on almost priest-like vantage points on a psychedelic drug that I firmly believe should be used only in ceremonial contexts and should not be perverted by indiscriminate cultural appropriation. This is a very special journey to go on and one that has many more elements to it than just the ingestion of the sacred vine.

Two of my favorite books on the topic are *The Fellowship of the River* by Dr. Joe Tafur and *Listening to Ayahuasca* by Rachel Harris. Both are beautiful tales of a metamorphosis that saw a Western medical doctor, Tafur, and a child of a '60s psychologist, Harris, see their work and lives through an entirely different lens after spending extensive time with both the medicine and the Indigenous tribes that serve them.

Tafur recounted his ancestral reconnection that was lost before taking Ayahuasca. He said, "In 2007 I took my first trip to Peru with Keyvan. I had my first Ayahuasca experience, and then I had two more very profound ceremonies on that visit as well. Each time the experience was more familiar. After the third ceremony, it was time to go. I wept that day. I wept in gratitude. I felt like those ceremonies had brought me 'back' to a connection with the South American soil. Even though I was born in the United States, my spirit had always felt somehow displaced. The Shipibos had somehow reconnected me to my roots and to the Earth. I did not realize how much I was aching for that connection."

Of all the compounds that I have studied, Ayahuasca seems to have a quality to it that doesn't just connect us to Godhead but that also reconnects us to our lineages that lie within and have somehow gotten lost due to the frenzied pace and disconnection of modern life. I've never been one to get too curious about where my seed came from, but upon listening to the plant teachers in the vine, I've been able to feel more connected to the earth and my origin story—and that's from minimal use of Ayahuasca. I suspect that if I ever feel called to go back to Grandmother Aya (as it's referred to by the Shipibo tribe of Peru), I can learn even more about who I am and where I come from.

The immense rise in popularity of Ayahuasca in the West has done for psychedelics in the twenty-first century what LSD did for them in the 1960s. Countless Western seekers from all walks of life have ventured down to the jungles and come back as if they've been touched by a disembodied spark of divinity. There is something about the ceremonial integrity of the actual use of the drug that has created a path for it to stay free from much of the stigma that typical counterculture drug takers receive. Its efficacy at treating trauma with veterans and its inherent ability to treat other illnesses that the Western medical model hasn't been able to is also opening up huge research avenues to the drug's potential.

Let's take a brief look at what exactly Ayahuasca is and how it's made. It's a fascinating process that demonstrates the beauty that occurs when humans tune into nature, listen to their ecosystem, and use the resources around them to heal and forge a deeper connection to their natural habitat.

Ayahuasca is a traditional psychoactive brew used in spiritual and religious ceremonies by Indigenous peoples in the Amazon basin. It's typically prepared by combining two main ingredients: the *Banisteriopsis caapi* vine and the leaves of the *Psychotria viridis* or other related plants containing DMT. How these Indigenous peoples managed to find these two separate plants to combine and create Ayahuasca among the countless species within the Amazon region is still a testament to traditional Indigenous sciences.

The preparation process involves several steps:

1. **Selecting the plants:** The *Banisteriopsis caapi* vine (also known as the Ayahuasca vine) is usually chosen for its MAOI properties. The *Psychotria viridis* leaves or other DMT-containing plants provide the hallucinogenic component.

2. **Cleaning and processing:** The vine and leaves are cleaned, often stripped of any unwanted parts, and sometimes pounded or crushed to facilitate extraction.

3. **Brewing:** The vine and leaves are combined in a large pot or cauldron with water. Sometimes additional plant materials might be added, depending on the specific traditional practices.

4. **Cooking:** The mixture is then boiled for several hours, often under the guidance of an experienced brewer. The length of boiling time can vary, and the process is believed to allow the active compounds to infuse into the liquid.

5. **Straining and cooling:** Once boiled, the liquid is strained to remove the plant material, resulting in a thick, muddy-looking brew. Afterward, it's left to cool.

The preparation of Ayahuasca involves a combination of plants containing psychoactive compounds that, when combined, create a brew that looks more like a purple sludge than like tea. The *Banisteriopsis caapi* vine contains MAOIs, which prevent the breakdown of DMT by enzymes in the stomach, allowing the DMT from the leaves to become orally active. The end result is a powerful psychoactive experience that when ingested can bring you face to face with the ancient teachers that live within the plants. The Shipibo tribe of Peru literally believe that the plants are our teachers and they are here to show us how to live in equanimity with the world around us.

They don't drink the tea to just float idly in the colorful visions and sacred geometry; they go there to do serious work. And that begins weeks before the drug is actually consumed with a process referred to as a "dieta," which is a pre-journey purification regimen that includes fasting, sexual abstinence, and a reduction in medical consumption that is aimed at cleansing the physical vessel to allow for the drug's magic to land with as much integrity as possible.

In the mid-1800s, Richard Spruce and Alexander von Humboldt were two of the first European explorers to encounter the Ayahuasca decoction. These early explorers reported hearing tales of the beverage's magical effects: stories of visions, "out-of-body travel," predictions of the future, location of lost objects, and contact with the dead. However, even with encounters by European colonists, the use of the drug didn't gain much traction outside of South America until Terence McKenna reintroduced it to the West in the 1980s and proclaimed its transcendental potential during his popular public talks. Most explorers, colonists, and even early twentieth-century botanists tended to otherize its use and label it as an exotic or primitive ritual.

Pre-Ayahuasca Journey Questions to Ask Yourself

1. Why do you want to use Ayahuasca in the first place? Are you clear about your intentions? Do you feel that taking Ayahuasca is in alignment with realizing your highest sense of self?

---

2. Ayahuasca is best left in the hands of Indigenous healers. Have you done your research and selected a healer or Ayahuasca retreat center that is both credible and safe?

3. Ayahuasca is incredibly potent and relentless. Are you ready to surrender to what's being shown to you rather than try to control the experience?

4. Describe any fears, mental or physical, that you have around taking Ayahuasca.

5. Are you in good health and feel that you can withstand the intensity of Ayahuasca? If not, be honest about it and recognize that this medicine might not be right for you. This includes any psychiatric medications that you may be on. Do not downplay the severity of these contra-indicators.

6. What is your integration plan? What are you going to do in the hours and days afterward?

Ayahuasca, LSD, mushrooms, MDMA, and short-acting DMT are all powerful psychotropic medicines that can change the very nature of who you are. Exploring your mind, body, and soul with the aid of these drugs is not for everyone. Some of us just aren't ready for the multitude of visions that these drugs will show us, while others should wait until better circumstances present themselves.

The drugs I discussed in this chapter are ones that I've had the most experience with, but they do not make a complete list of psychedelic drugs that are present in today's psychonaut cabinet. The mescaline family of compounds, which include synthetic mescaline and organic plants like San Pedro and peyote, have incredibly rich traditions that are being kept alive in organizations like the Native American Church. And there's ketamine, which has become wildly popular recently (almost too much) in treating depression and other mental health issues. Because ketamine is legal, there are clinics in nearly every major US city that serve those who need alternative approaches to their mental health issues.

Sasha Shulgin, the brilliant chemist who synthesized MDMA, didn't stop at just that one drug. His book *PiHKAL: A Chemical Love Story*, written with his wife Ann, documents the hundreds (yes, hundreds) of other phenethylamine molecules that he created in his humble laboratory in Northern California. Most of these never saw the light of day in terms of being used on humans, but a few did. Namely 2C-B (4-bromo-2,5-dimethoxyphenethylamine), which in my experience acts a little like MDMA, a little like LSD, and a whole lot like nothing else you've ever experienced. The Shulgins' lifelong love story and quest to further understand the workings of the human mind and the potential of new interpersonal communications that can happen under the influence of these drugs are testaments to the ever-expanding world of psychedelic-assisted exploration and therapy.

The drugs I've included in this chapter are certainly the most common psychedelics on the scene today, but I suspect that in the next one hundred years, we will see an outpouring of new molecules that will expand the human relationship with psychedelic substances. There is an entire industry currently blooming that is refining and testing new drugs that are not only safe but are designed to seamlessly graft onto the human brain. Simultaneously, more and more people are becoming aware and increasingly respectful of the age-old Indigenous traditions that have used these drugs for thousands of years. There's no doubt that the world of psychedelics, both natural and synthetic, is just getting started.

3

The Medicalization Model

A Cautionary Partnership

Flash back fifteen years ago to the medical cannabis movement in California, prior to the recreational laws currently in effect, and you might remember the scene at Venice Beach on any given day. There were countless salespeople dressed up in wild green costumes ushering pretty much anyone who "needed" a medical card into a doctor's office. Upon paying your $50, a "doctor" would give you a medical card for cannabis just as long as you verbally confirmed that you suffered from a myriad of medical conditions ranging from depression and anxiety to sleeping problems. No real due diligence was performed, and it became generally accepted among the California stoner population that if you wanted legal cannabis, all you had to do was feign a medical issue and you'd be granted access. It was a legal workaround that ended up becoming a mockery of legitimate medical use.

A current model exists within the ketamine clinic ecosystem. Yes, there are many ketamine clinics with top-rate psychologically trained administrators who are indeed there to provide relief for those deeply afflicted with mental health conditions. But there are just as many clinics where you can walk in, spend ten minutes with an intake counselor, tell them that you're depressed, and they will have you hooked up to a ketamine IV in minutes. Not only is this an abuse of the mental health system, but it also creates room for the massively profitable ketamine clinic business to thrive with no concern for actual mental health treatment.

If we strictly follow the medicalized model for the classic psychedelics like psilocybin and MDMA, we could potentially see the same thing: countless seekers finding a therapist who administers these medicines and circumvents mental health issues for the sake of providing a high-cost mystical experience to the curious. Think of it as high-priced psychedelic tourism controlled by the wealthy.

We are also seeing a tsunami wave of psychotherapists rushing to get "certified" to administer psychedelics, even though they have as little as one or two personal session experiences themselves, which in turn makes the practice of administering these medicines sterile and void of the mystical transformation that can potentially occur. How can one person create a container for a profound mystical experience when they have only intellectual knowledge of it themselves? The psychedelic experience does not happen by osmosis. It is a deeply personal, potentially mystical, and wholly transformative experience that needs support from all parts of an interpersonal structure that is deeply immersed in these occurrences.

In the end, I believe that the upsides outweigh the negatives in the medical model, for both those suffering from mental health issues and those taking advantage of the system. The result is that a safe container and well-thought-out psychosocial "set" will be available, thus reducing the risks associated with casual psychedelic use—when done right. Proper education, almost exhaustive prep work, and rigid post-journey integration are all cornerstones of the psychedelic-assisted therapy model. This also means that voyagers will have more meaningful single journeys and won't be as seduced into the trap of overuse. This is a good thing.

Still, the horrors of so-called "conscious corporations" are poised to set themselves up to rake in massive profits, all while creating an access system for those who can afford it and doing nothing to keep the Indigenous traditions alive, thriving, and respected. If the future of psychedelics ends up in a sterile, therapeutic setting accompanied by high-cost access and the federal drug laws around recreational use stay put, then psychedelic advocates and researchers have accomplished very little as a community.

There is mixed opinion held by many in power within the psychedelic space. Many argue that in order to provide safe and effective access to psychedelics, their use must be regulated and supervised by medical professionals, while others like myself argue that we should raise a cautionary flag because of the potential in creating new power systems that govern these therapeutic bodies.

Misunderstanding Decriminalization

In October 2023, California governor Gavin Newsom vetoed a bill that would have decriminalized magic mushrooms and other psychedelic drugs in the state of California. In his veto statement to Senate Bill 58, he said, "California should immediately begin work to set up regulated treatment guidelines—replete with dosing information, therapeutic guidelines, rules to prevent exploitation during guided treatments, and medical clearance of no underlying psychoses. Unfortunately, this bill would decriminalize possession prior to these guidelines going into place, and I cannot sign it."

Newsom's words here are very deliberate and very telling. While he did veto this bill, he did it with the focus being on the medicalized application of psychedelics being of the utmost priority. It wasn't an outright dismissal of the transformational power of psychedelics. It was a cautious embrace of the tremendous potential to help solve the mental health crisis that is currently affecting the country.

At first glance, one might think that his statement is optimistic and open-minded. It's not ridden with typical politician hysteria around psychedelics, and that's a good thing. The problem with it is that it reinforces the narrative that psychedelics are headed toward widespread acceptance only for the treatment of mental health issues and not as part of the larger discussion around cognitive liberty and the failed War on Drugs. The reality is that a growing number of Californians (and people in other states) are currently using these medicines for reasons that may include spiritual growth, Indigenous ritual and celebration, and possibly even safe personal recreational situations. The fact that Newsom's comments don't even address the reformation of the failed War on Drugs is tone deaf to what the current landscape looks like, instead projecting to a not fully realized vision for how it might look in the future.

Senator Scott Wiener (D-California), the bill's author said, "This is a setback for the huge number of Californians—including combat veterans and first responders—who are safely using and benefiting from these non-addictive substances and who will now continue to be classified as criminals under California law."

What we have to understand about decriminalization bills that are popping up all around the country is that they are not the same thing as legalization bills. Decriminalization and legalization are two very different things. Decriminalization only means that the people who already somehow have obtained these currently illegal drugs can now possess them in low quantities without fear of prosecution. It does nothing for the buying and selling of these unregulated drugs and how they make their way into the marketplace. The underground commerce of illegal drugs is a multibillion-dollar industry that gives power to shady groups, like cartels and gangs, and fuels a civil war of citizens versus law enforcement. Decriminalization actually does very little to end the most violent and deadly part of the War on Drugs. It is merely a ceremonial gesture to the millions of Americans who are already using these drugs that tells them that they are not criminals and that the current system is broken. However, these efforts are a very simple first step in the admission that the madness needs to end.

What we have here is a schism within the psychedelic community. For decades, crusaders who were fighting to combat the draconian antidrug laws have made strides in getting the general public (and politicians) to understand that the War on Drugs has failed while simultaneously educating the public around the newfound efficacy that psychedelics have uncovered in treating mental health issues. The psychedelic renaissance ushered in a tremendous wave of hope through the groundbreaking clinical trials at various institutions like Johns Hopkins, NYU, and the Department of Veterans Affairs via MAPS.

The two paths were linked together to make good on objectives that had many boxes to check. Redefining mental health treatment and criminal justice reform were two sides of the same coin and needed to be talked about in unison so those opposed could understand the bigger picture and get reeducated on decades of false narratives. So when we see a senior level politician like Gov. Gavin Newsom emphasizing only one part of the story around psychedelic drug reform, it creates even more misunderstanding around how these drugs are being used collectively. However, it also amazes me that he is aware of the therapeutic potential of psychedelic drugs and is even talking about granular details like dosage guidelines and safety. So it's not all bad.

But how did we get here? How did the medicalized use of psychedelics in the form of psychedelic-assisted therapy become the predominant conversation in their current evolution?

The MAPS Effect

Before Doblin started MAPS in 1986, the supply of MDMA could not meet the demand of party-going kids because of the chemical complexity in creating pure MDMA. As a result, untold amounts of impure versions of the drug flooded the market and it became known as Molly and, most commonly, Ecstasy. These pressed-pill nightmares of unreliable purity, often with dangerous additives, were instantly problematic and led to a large number of poor physical reactions to taking the drug, which resulted in medical emergencies for some and perhaps most importantly a new wave of propaganda around the safety and usefulness of MDMA. Just like a repeat of LSD in the '60s, the drug left research laboratories and quickly became criminalized when used by the general public, thus outlawing the potential for therapy and research.

The good news is after that, Doblin quickly started MAPS and began a mission that at first seemed impossible. Not only did Doblin see the potential to treat PTSD firsthand with MDMA, he took it a step further and asked the question, "What population suffers most from PTSD and is ignored?" The answers to that question are veterans and first responders.

When Doblin said he was going to go into the front door of the Pentagon to ask for permission to work with PTSD-ridden veterans using MDMA-assisted therapy as the treatment, the nascent psychedelic community of the late '80s and early '90s thought he was mad. Not only did the mission seem impossible, but it was also a sweeping insult to the old guards of the counterculture. How could this new upstart psychedelic crusader want to work with our enemy? The military? Madness!

It's a good thing that all the old hippies who were attached to keeping psychedelics part of whatever was left of the '60s were wrong. Not only did Doblin succeed in working with veterans via the MAPS-sponsored PTSD clinical trials, but he also ushered in a whole new era of legitimate psychedelic research that countless institutions, scientists, doctors, and therapists would follow for the next thirty years. Psychedelic-assisted therapy was back and here to stay.

Rick Doblin and MAPS are of course some of the leaders in this movement, but others like Dr. Roland Griffiths at Johns Hopkins, Dr. Charles Grob at UCLA, and Dr. Anthony Bossis at NYU followed with their own research and published breakthrough therapy models and results that helped lay the foundation for not only mental health treatment but for a far more disciplined approach to using psychedelics as a whole. What I mean by that is that the model for psychedelic-assisted therapy—which includes rigorous screening, extra care with set and setting, and a blueprint for mapping out one's intentions—left the research setting and became the de facto standard for anyone who wants to use psychedelics. When I hear even the most novice psychonaut who is venturing into using these drugs for the first time talk about preparation, set, and setting and ask about the risks in such a curious and disciplined way, I am thrilled that so much care is being put into going on this adventure. The days of dropping five hundred micrograms of LSD and running around at a Grateful Dead concert hoping for the best are far less common than it used to be.

Dr. Griffiths, who headed up the psychedelic studies department at Johns Hopkins, recently passed away and left behind a legacy of successful research and fastidious attention to data and detail that is so important. Because of the legitimacy of Johns Hopkins, his work helped change the minds of so many who were shut off from even discussing the potential of psychedelic-assisted therapy.

The treatment-resistant depression study at Johns Hopkins, in particular, is a go-to case study that I like to refer to because of its effectiveness and the nature of it being so accessible for anyone interested in the method. Twenty-four people who had a long-term documented history of depression, most of whom experienced persisting symptoms for approximately two years, underwent two five-hour psilocybin sessions under the direction of the researchers, with four-week follow-ups.

"The magnitude of the effect we saw was about four times larger than what clinical trials have shown for traditional antidepressants on the market," said Dr. Alan Davis, adjunct assistant professor of psychiatry and behavioral sciences at Johns Hopkins University School of Medicine. "Because most other depression treatments take weeks or months to work and may have undesirable effects, this could be a game changer if these findings hold up in future 'gold-standard' placebo-controlled clinical trials."

Griffiths went on to say of the study, "Because there are several types of major depressive disorders that may result in variation in how people respond to treatment, I was surprised that most of our study participants found the psilocybin treatment to be effective."

Over in Switzerland, Peter Gasser, head of the Swiss Medical Society for Psycholytic Therapy—which he joined after his own therapist-administered LSD experience—has only recently begun to discuss his research into the possible therapeutic effects of LSD on the intense anxiety experienced by patients with life-threatening diseases such as cancer. The $190,000 study approved by Swiss medical authorities was almost entirely funded by MAPS.

Begun in 2008, the study treated twelve patients (eight with LSD, four with placebo) who found the experience aided them emotionally, and none experienced panic reactions or other untoward events. One patient, Udo Schulz, told the German weekly *Der Spiegel* that the therapy with LSD helped him overcome anxious feelings after being diagnosed with stomach cancer, and the experience with the drug aided his reentry into the workplace.

There are countless peer-reviewed case studies like the ones mentioned here that have created a wellspring of a database that not only shows that these drugs are effective in treating various mental health conditions but are in fact safe when used wisely. If you head over to psychedelicsurvey.com or Google Scholar, you can read these studies for yourself. You'll be amazed at how many there have been and how successful the outcomes are.

The halo effect that this has had on the stuffy naysayers is simply amazing. I find it head scratching that former governor of Texas and Trump cabinet member Rick Perry is advocating for treating veterans' PTSD with MDMA. That is something I never dreamed would happen in my lifetime.

Bestsellers and Op-Eds

But even so, there is still a great divide among those who have had their lives changed thanks to psychedelics and their desire to have them more widely available to others. For example, take Michael Pollan's wildly popular book *How to Change Your Mind*. Most of the book's focus is on the mental health benefits of psychedelics and institutional acceptance, and encourages a very bureaucratic approach to rolling them out to a larger population. What seems to be absent is a nuanced dialogue about the rich, magical, mystical tapestries that psychedelics can induce, which is understandable given Pollan is a relatively new psychonaut with only a few psychedelic experiences of his own. On the other hand, I am acutely aware of how many lives that book touched and how many minds were changed thanks to Pollan's very balanced narrative and his already accepted credibility as a writer. There's no doubt the book helped move the needle in a positive direction.

Even after the success of the book and Pollan's own newfound role as a psychedelic expert, he has been vocal about putting the brakes on legalization in favor of more research within the medicalization framework. In the 2019 *New York Times* op-ed piece entitled "Not So Fast on Psychedelic Mushrooms," the subtitle said it all: "Psilocybin has a lot of potential as medicine, but we don't know enough about it yet to legalize it."

That to me was one of the most offensive op-eds ever given voice to the subject of psychedelics. The implication is that the scientific method is all that matters, and the previous multi-millennia of Indigenous and ceremonial use does not hold the same weight as modern science's investigation into its use. And to suggest that psilocybin is only a "medicine" that should be used under the supervision of licensed clinicians is the very essence of corporate gatekeeping. This is just another example of why it takes so long to truly change people's hearts, souls, and minds about what it means to let go of control and offer people the right to think for themselves. I certainly don't feel compelled to be arrogant enough to think I can tell anyone what is or isn't the right way for them to further their hunger for existential knowledge.

Corpa-Delic Culture's Insatiable Appropriation

In October 2022, the *New York Times* published yet another extensive piece on psychedelics, this time aimed at exposing the complicated web of new start-ups: "With Promise of Legalization, Psychedelic Companies Joust Over Future Profits" with the subtitle "Cash rich start-ups are filing scores of patent claims on hallucinogens like magic mushrooms. Researchers and patient advocates worry high prices will make the therapies unaffordable."

UK-based Compass Pathways has set itself up to be the first legal provider of psilocybin, having recently launched a massive clinical study across Europe and North America to test the drug as a treatment for depression. In 2018, Compass's psilocybin received "breakthrough therapy designation" from the FDA, meaning the study will be fast-tracked through the drug-development process. Compass is making an aggressive bid to patent techniques for synthesizing psilocybin-like compounds. By creating their own synthetic version of psilocybin, which can be patented because it only has a small difference in molecular structure, they have paved the way for a profit-driven monopoly whose primary objective is profit over the dissemination of a truly magical healing experience.

For those of us in the know, we are well aware that psilocybin, the active ingredient in magic mushrooms, is a compound that cannot be patented due to it being a natural derivative that grows just about anywhere in the world. Plant medicine allies see the adoption and subsequent patent of synthetic psilocybin as a move that defeats the whole purpose of these drugs making their way into the mainstream treatment of mental health disorders. It's a move that creates overregulation while also paving the way for someone, perhaps Compass, to make millions in profits from a treatment that has no one owner or control over it.

The concept of "set and setting" was first theorized in the 1964 book *The Psychedelic Experience* by Timothy Leary, Richard Alpert (later Ram Dass), and Ralph Metzner. The idea was to create some parameters for how adults who wished to alter their consciousness with the use of psychedelics could do so safely and effectively. It was meant as a loose set of guidelines that anyone could adapt with their own unique flavor in conducting a psychedelic session and/or ritual. Compass has tried to file a worldwide patent on the entire psychedelic process, which includes set and setting and the medicine itself. How can you patent "set and setting"? Well, they've tried to patent the technique of using an eye mask and sitting on a couch during a session. Really.

Andrew Jacobs wrote in *The Times*: "One patent application for psilocybin therapy claimed its treatment rooms were unique because they featured 'muted colors,' high-fidelity sound systems, and cozy furniture. Another sought exclusivity on a therapist reassuringly holding the hand of a patient. Then there's the patent seeking a monopoly on nearly all methods of delivering the drug to patients, including vaginally and rectally." Such egregious patent claims "have provoked howls of derision from some scientists and patient advocates, who warn that corporate efforts to profit from existing drugs, like psilocybin, LSD, and MDMA, could chill academic research and throttle public access by making new therapies prohibitively expensive."

To me, it's laughable that anyone thinks they can patent and define a psychedelic medicine experience that has its roots in Indigenous wisdom and tradition. Just because the modern spin of psychedelic-assisted therapy is added to the mix does not mean that it's a new modality. I'd agree that when used in a therapeutic setting, the systems in place need to have some form of regulation and safety protocols to make sure that a) the facilitators doing this work are qualified and b) no further harm will come to the patient. But I don't subscribe to the fact that certain newly powerful companies can be left to pave the way for complete control of the treatment. This is dangerous and offensive. It is also misleading to the public at large. Many newer psychedelic curiosity seekers are under the impression that the administration of psychedelics belongs to the power structures of the medical establishment. Anyone familiar with Indigenous use surely knows this isn't true.

Compass Pathways is just one of many new start-ups making their way onto the scene. And not all of them are driven by capitalist intentions; many are set up to provide education and infrastructure support to a brand-new industry that does indeed need some guidance in this brave new world of psychedelic exploration. This is the very embodiment of treachery when billionaires like Peter Thiel invest in something new that they don't fully understand. Psychedelic healing is so popular that I can see why the venture capital community sees the gold rush more than they do the empathy or the transformational experience.

Pros and Cons of Medicalization

The medical application of psychedelics for the veteran population is yet another paradox. In the early '90s when Doblin said treating vets with PTSD was a primary mission for MAPS, everyone thought it couldn't be done. Thirty years later, not only is MDMA on the verge of completing an FDA-approved Phase 3 clinical trial (which means it will be legal in clinical settings), the success with the veteran population has turned psychedelic-assisted therapy into a mainstream treatment. The default association of psychedelics with hippies and wild-eyed outlaw researchers has come to an end, and an entire industry has formed around the culture, creating what I like to refer to as "corpa-delic" culture.

It's important to examine the pros and cons of the rise in the medical applications of psychedelic use because it reveals what the psychedelic community is doing well and where the red flags are. The basic premise is that when you take a method that has its roots in culturally significant Indigenous practices (psychedelic healing) and juxtapose it against a capitalistic backdrop, you are left with a well-intentioned juggernaut that is fraught with the perils of money, profit, high barriers to access, and players who are in it for the wrong reasons.

Because of its rise in popularity, nearly all newcomers to the space have been made aware of these drugs due to the success they have found in mental health circles. In the last five years, I have had more people come to me seeking help who have read headlines in the *New York Times*, read Michael Pollan's book, or know a veteran whose life has been saved thanks to psychedelics. But those who find me who are aware of only the clinical aspects seem to lack an understanding of the holistic effect psychedelics will have on their lives. They think this is somehow a magic bullet with pharmacological properties (and not the deep inner work) that will heal them.

These are but a few of the pros and cons I see within the rise of the medicalized application of psychedelic drugs.

The Pros

Redefining mental health: From both a pragmatic and educational standpoint, the research and clinical trials on how psychedelics have affected the mental health crisis around the world can't be ignored. Suddenly this crisis, which has affected nearly everyone directly or indirectly, has a new glimmer of hope. The chance for real suffering to end is a strong possibility.

Data: For whatever reason, the US especially is data driven. In the age of Big Data, it seems that once people see the numbers, it helps change their minds. The endless research done with psychedelics in the last twenty years has created more data than we know what to do with.

High efficacy: More in line with data, but the fact the efficacy rates are so high has helped change the minds of so many and prove empirically that these are no longer fringe treatments. For instance, the Phase 3 MAPS PTSD-MDMA clinical trials have a high success rate, with 71 percent of participants who underwent therapy with the combination of MDMA no longer meeting the DSM-5 criteria for PTSD.

Safety: Clinical settings have shown that when these drugs are used safely, they are in fact not any more dangerous than other pharmaceuticals. Yes, they still carry risks but not at the rate that the DEA led us to believe. This also translates into recreational users asking more questions about the risks than going into it blindly. I haven't heard anyone say, "If I take LSD, will I never come back?" in a long, long time. The narratives around psychedelic use have changed in a good way and have permeated the mainstream healing world and pop culture. Thanks to highly supervised clinical trials that are rigorous around drug purity, patient suitability, and set and setting, we now can say that the risks surrounding using these drugs are far less extraordinary than previously thought.

The Cons

High barrier for entry: It's safe to say that high costs were not an intentional mistake when setting out to legalize psychedelic-assisted therapy. For instance, if the MAPS MDMA protocol became legal today, it would cost anywhere from $10,000 to $15,000 to do the three sessions in a legal supervised manner. Having insurance cover it or not is not the point. This is emblematic of how an amazing breakthrough therapy introduced into the mainstream mental health system is not only fraught with regulation and bureaucracy but is also unattainable for countless people who could benefit from it.

Elitism: Because of the high price point, a certain air of elitism has taken over the conversation regarding access to these treatments. If only the wealthy can afford it, then what have we really accomplished?

Sterile and void of mystical properties: This is perhaps my most pressing issue with the rise of the medicalization movement. Because psychedelics have now defaulted to being a clinical treatment in the minds of so many, the treatment itself has become more reminiscent of a visit to a doctor's office than a trip into the mystical space of wonder and magic. Many clinicians who are now getting into this space are putting far too much emphasis on the cognitively based therapy part of the process and are not prepping users for the journey into the unknown. There are parts of the psychedelic experience that aren't meant to be understood in how and why they work. There's a certain element of mystery in why these spirit molecules unlock a sense of oneness in the individual. So when I hear an upstart psychedelic therapist talking only about the pharmacology of these compounds and not the sense of mystical awareness that might occur, I cringe.

The over-medicalization promotes the vast sterilization of the psychedelic experience. Trying to erase the mystical DNA from psychedelics is like trying to erase heat from the sun. Sometimes we can't control nature or explain its vast and unspoken properties.

Psychedelic exceptionalism: This is apparent in Gov. Newsom's comments. The idea that psychedelics are somehow so special that they don't tie into the general War on Drugs and don't fit into the basic idea that one should have the right to change their consciousness as they see fit is alarming. Yes, psychedelics work on the mind differently than, say, heroin, but that doesn't mean the psychedelic community should distance itself from the nature of drug use as a whole. Columbia University professor Dr. Carl Hart wrote in his book *Drug Use for Grown-Ups: Chasing Liberty in the Land of Fear*, "Clearly, many people consume psychoactive substances 'in the pursuit of happiness,' a right the government was established to secure, to protect. So why then is our current government arresting one million Americans each year for possessing drugs? Why are so many drug users hiding in the closet? This reality does not align with the spirit of the Declaration."

If you dig further into Dr. Hart's book and work, you'll find more rationale on why viewing psychedelics as an elitist paradigm distant from other recreational drug users is dangerous and the product of an elite agenda.

Systemic replacement: We all agree that the mental health system is broken. No one can argue with that. Millions have been left with no effective solutions or institutions to turn to and are suffering. The rise of psychedelic-assisted therapy has largely been a commentary on the failure of such systems (i.e., the Department of Veterans Affairs's treatment of vets), but as corpa-delic culture rises, I am beginning to see that a large part of the community is simply replacing one system with another.

The Naysayers and Disgruntled Detractors

Psychedelic research in a clinical setting continues to surprise even the most ardent cynics in the twenty-first century. Countless trial participants have been amazed at the turnaround they have experienced at the hands of psychedelic medicines like psilocybin and MDMA. Yet, in early 2024, there have been a couple of noteworthy setbacks that, to me, speak to the idea that mainstream medical organizations are still looking for ways to take away from the success. The fact remains that if you stare at anything long enough, you will begin to see its imperfections and will start to find something wrong with it. The same applies to psychedelic research.

I firmly reside in the camp that most of the psychedelic research done in the last ten years has opened up a tremendous window into the understanding of the human brain, our perception of reality, and new ways in which we can learn to heal issues that are plaguing our society. However, I am not a research fellow or a hardcore academic who spends my time poring over the granular details of every single peer-reviewed study and faction of data presented on using psychedelic drugs as the primary method for change. My tendency to see things from the larger cultural perspective affects my bias. For instance, the sheer positive impact that Johns Hopkins has had on the medical community at large for even creating a psychedelic studies department far outweighs the unfavorable aspects of the data. I've met countless doctors, nurses, and citizens who have stated that the weight of Hopkins's psychedelic research has opened up their mind to learn more.

Or take the MAPS PTSD Phase 3 trials for instance, which state that 71.2 percent of participants who received MDMA-assisted therapy, compared to 47.6 percent of participants receiving placebo plus therapy, no longer met DSM-5 diagnostic criteria for PTSD at the end of the study. The 71 percent efficacy rate is an extraordinary indicator that these medicines may hold a therapeutic potential that we are only beginning to fully understand. Once MDMA becomes legal as a prescription drug to treat PTSD, the approach to that form of psychedelic-assisted therapy will become more mature and tailored to address trauma in populations that we aren't even aware of yet. The best is yet to come.

Yet, even with success rates that high, there are still potential gaps in the research that say the "clinical evidence is insufficient." On March 27, 2023, just a short few months before the FDA was set to administer their final approval of MDMA as a legal therapeutic option for those suffering from PTSD, nonprofit health care think tank Institute for Clinical and Economic Review (ICER) published a report that was critical of the Lykos (formerly MAPS PBC) Phase 3 MDMA clinical trials. ICER Chief Medical Officer David Rind said, "While MDMA-AP may be a promising therapy for PTSD . . . functional unblinding in the clinical trials and additional concerns around trial design and conduct leave many uncertainties about the balance of benefits and harms."

Josh Hardman, the editor at *Psychedelic Alpha*, wrote: "In short: ICER is pessimistic regarding the level of clinical evidence provided by Lykos Therapeutics, highlighting various concerns that range from trial design and conduct issues through to potential ethical and safety problems. While the organization is generally relaying concerns it has heard from parties with 'firsthand' and 'secondhand' experience or knowledge of the trials, it's hard not to see certain sections as scathing."

Again, it's hard (if not impossible) to make cognitive bias a factor in trying to understand these findings. I have witnessed firsthand the tremendous effects MDMA has had in the reduction of PTSD in vets and sexual abuse survivors. Also, my personal experience with MDMA in an intentional setting has offered me a tremendous amount of relief around the trauma I experienced as a substance abuse addict who experienced homelessness and physical assault. I am not a scientist in the sense that the data I've collected is nothing more than personal experiences and stories heard from others. It is not data that can fit neatly into a spreadsheet or any other collection tool. For me, actually seeing the change in others is the greatest data I can ever come across.

It's my understanding that the MAPS/Lykos trials have indeed seen efficacy rates as high as they claim, but yes, the negative results have been downplayed in the spirit of focusing on the positive and not the negative. Was this a wise approach for the greater good? From a scientific perspective, I can see how this is alarming, and organizations like MAPS/Lykos should be fully transparent in all the data, even the negative experiences. For instance, during the MAPS/Lykos Phase 2 clinical trials, there was a treatment team out of Canada that sexually abused and manipulated a vulnerable trial patient under the influence of MDMA. The video of the session in question is public and quite alarming—serious trigger warning. I do think MAPS should have been much more vocal in their disgust of that event and should usher in more community-based discussions on how this can be avoided in the future. We can learn so much as a community from our mistakes if we talk about them openly and with full transparency.

Still, I wonder what agendas organizations like ICER have in being naysayers for the advancement of psychedelic research. Is the data actually flawed? Or are they representative of an old-school medical establishment that does not want to see psychedelics have a place in the mainstreaming of mental health treatment? Could it be that, simply put, some people just aren't ready for it? I suspect that's part of it. What I find so interesting about psychedelic research is that much of the data acquired is in actuality very hard to quantify. How do you quantify an increase in compassion toward the self? How do you quantify a reduction in self-limiting belief systems? How do you quantify a mystical experience? The latter has been shown to be increasingly difficult for the scientific community to get its head around because it challenges the very notion of the scientific method.

And sure enough on August 9, 2024, the FDA followed the advice of the AdComm panel and the negative ICER report and did not approve MDMA for the treatment of PTSD. This has been the primary mission of MAPS (and now Lykos) for the past two decades, so no doubt it was a blow to everyone involved. There's no question that the work will continue and that at some point, psychedelics will find a place within the medical establishment.

How and why the FDA did not end up approving MDMA for clinical trials they helped design is a Hollywood melodrama of a story that would make for a scintillating Netflix series. Nirvan Mullick, a filmmaker who is making a documentary on Rick Doblin, summed up the situation by saying, "Everyone had such faith in the efficacy, which was proven in clinical trials and published in *Nature*, one of the most respected peer-reviewed scientific journals. Everyone was confident that the FDA would follow the science, especially as the FDA had signed off on the design of this study after a lengthy special review. I think everyone underestimated how quickly the FDA's fears could be triggered by an exaggerated sensationalist smear campaign orchestrated by anti-capitalist Psymposia (radical activists who don't want psychedelics commercialized) and then magnified by ICER (a special interest group that works with the insurance industry to advise on drug prices). It was a shocking collapse and failure that will deprive over 13 million Americans suffering from PTSD from a treatment shown to be twice as effective as any existing treatment. And you don't have to keep taking it forever! It was so upsetting and shows how deeply flawed the FDA regulatory process is."

It's deeply sad to me that there is a vocal minority within the psychedelic community that wants to see others fail, create disinformation, and take half-truths and turn them into an anarchic style of chaos. The MAPS/Lykos clinical trials were far from perfect, but if the FDA approved MDMA, there would have been tens of thousands of Americans who could have immediately benefited from the treatment. To deny them that right to heal in favor of pushing an anti-medicalization model is both self-interested and short-sighted. It's important to remember that medicalization leads to a change in policy, which can slowly change the tide in our draconian drug laws. There are certainly some bad actors on the medicalization stage—those who want to control the entire psychedelic rollout and turn it into a monopoly—but this was not one of those cases. Everyone loses here.

Are True Believers a Bad Thing?

On March 21, 2024, *New York Times* reporter Brendan Borrell published a head-scratching piece on the legacy of Roland Griffiths, the dearly departed maverick psychedelic researcher at Johns Hopkins. It labeled him "a true believer," and that alone puts his data into question. Over time, Griffiths became somewhat of a legend in the psychedelic community, not just for the research but also because he was unapologetic about his mystical leanings and personal experiences with psychedelics. Somehow, some people hold this against him and the tremendous work he did because it was indicative of a wild-eyed evangelist mystic reminiscent of days past. The *NYT* article said, "Some researchers have quietly questioned whether Dr. Griffiths, in his focus on the mystical realm, made some of the same mistakes that doomed the previous era of psychedelic science."

Matthew Johnson, a twenty-year collaborator of Griffiths, left Hopkins amid a wave of interpersonal tension and took it to the next level by saying of Griffiths, "Dr. Griffiths has run his psychedelic studies more like a 'new-age' retreat center, for lack of a better term, than a clinical research laboratory." That's very strong and charged language. Digging further into Johnson's critiques, the article stated,

"Dr. Griffiths acted like a 'spiritual leader,' the complaint said, 'infusing the research with religious symbolism and steering volunteers toward the outcome he wanted.'" What this means in real-world terms is that Griffiths placed statues of the Buddha in treatment rooms and was even heard to utter a "namaste" to trial participants now and then.

Think about that for a moment.

Is the scientific community that afraid of spirituality to the point that having a statue of the Buddha somehow threatens the integrity of the data? What's the alternative? Should psychedelic therapy rooms for clinical trials be stark white with nothing but a couch and some pretty flowers? Should the therapists enter the room dressed in a white lab coat with a clipboard, intent on treating the voyager like someone going in to have their gallbladder removed? Is there something unscientific by greeting the voyager with warmth and ensuring that their experience can lead to the most compassionate outcome possible?

It's bonkers to me that a leading psychedelic researcher is getting bashed posthumously for being sensitive to the fact that the psychedelic experience is mystical by default and that he wanted to ensure that the "setting" was conducive for a mystical outcome. This brings us back to the arrogance of the scientific method that decries any hint of encouraging mystical experiences into psychedelic data because it can't be quantified. Suggesting trials conducted like this are closer to "new-age retreat centers" highlights the vast expanse between cold and sterile scientific uses of psychedelics and the important Indigenous ceremonies that have been laying the foundation for all psychedelic use for the past several thousand years.

Both ICER's critique of the MAPS/Lykos trials and the Matt Johnson–led *NYT* hit piece on Roland Griffiths's legacy show us all that there will always be people and institutions within this revolution who will look for holes. Even if there are legitimate concerns to raise, what troubles me is the throwing the baby out with the bathwater tendency of those who do find flaws. As a community we all have work to do in adding transparency to when things go awry, especially when people are victimized by the hands of power-hungry therapists. But I remain confident that the magic of psychedelic healing is so powerful that the effectiveness can't help but rise to the top.

How We Move Forward with Medicalized Psychedelics

In order to roll out psychedelics safely, my thinking is that each subgenre of psychedelic culture should have a seat at the table, in which everyone can learn from each other. These include psychedelic therapists, psychedelic pharma companies, Indigenous healers, pro-decriminalization policy makers, and all-around drug war crusaders. For instance, newly enthused therapists who have moved into psychedelics can learn from Indigenous tribes' age-old ceremonial use of plant medicines and vice versa. There's a lot about mental health that healers can learn from empathetic and evolved psychologists, like Dr. Gabor Maté for instance.

And just because so many have gotten turned on to the modern psychedelic movement through mental health awareness doesn't mean that recreational users need to be looked at as the irresponsible undercurrent of users who might ruin it for everyone else. I know of countless underground psychedelic therapists and psychonauts who have explored these medicines and have come back as better people and practitioners. The fight for the original seed of cosmic crusading whose edict is "I have the right to change my consciousness as I see fit" can live alongside the need for safe and regulated access to psychedelic-assisted mental health treatment. They are not mutually exclusive.

Of course, it's wonderful that so many have found relief, but it's wrong to ignore and criminalize the millions of others who are using these drugs for purposes other than mental health issues. Mankind's hunger for setting forth on an epic hero's journey of self-inquiry, mystical exploration, and oneness is just as valid an intention as wanting to heal depression, anxiety, or PTSD. The sooner we learn to accept psychedelic compounds and their various valid uses, the sooner we create less judgment within the community (and outside of it), dissolve any warring factions, and highlight the need for criminal justice reform. However, I do admit that the process for changing the minds of the majority of naysayers on a topic like the use of psychedelic drugs takes time, patience, and a shift in social narrative. Having data that is based on health and wellness can create a halo effect that then seeps over into a broader acceptance of recreational use.

If you take the legalization of cannabis in California, you can see how this process might unfold. California became the first state to allow medicinal cannabis use when voters passed the Compassionate Use Act in 1996, and it wasn't until 2016 that it become legal for recreational use. In fact, in 2010, Proposition 10, which would have legalized recreational use, failed by a vote of 57 percent to 43 percent. It seems that voters simply needed more data to show that it was safe and effective before they went all in on the now ubiquitous cannabis shops that dot the state. I suspect that the same thing will happen with psychedelics. It's strange to me that most new individual awareness around psychedelics is based on their mental health benefits. I've also seen those same users want to continue their psychedelic explorations long after their clinical treatments are over. Once you pull back the curtain, you can't unsee it.

While I am critical of the over-medicalized application of psychedelics, I do see medicalized application as a means to an end. People like me don't need their minds changed. But people who are on the other side of the fence simply need to be reassured that these drugs aren't nearly as dangerous as they once thought and that they have a real benefit to mankind.

4

The Trauma in All of Us and How Psychedelics Can Revolutionize It

I f you take an honest look around the world today, it's easy to see that undiagnosed or unacknowledged trauma is influencing the state of the world and all who live in it. Today's world is smaller thanks to endless streams of media broadcasting an onslaught of death and disaster alongside cute animal videos on TikTok. Where good news ends and bad news begins is impossible to discern. We like to think we've become numb to the multitude of traumatic images we see in any given news cycle. But we haven't. They affect us. Even the constant consumption of mainstream media induces vicarious trauma for those viewing it.

These traumatic images are literal representations of all the pain and suffering that a record number of citizens in countries all over the globe are experiencing. Suicide rates are up in record numbers, anxiety levels are at an all-time high, and depression is being diagnosed at levels never before seen in modern history. There are many factors at work that are influencing trauma: economic woes, systemic racism, wealth inequality, discrimination of all kinds, and political divisions. And young people (women especially) are being fed social narratives around beauty standards and body types that have contributed to record highs in diagnosed eating disorders and school bullying. Whatever the reasons are for trauma manifesting into the psyche and nervous systems of our populations, the bigger problem is that most people aren't even aware that they are traumatized. And the problem after that is most of the available routes for healing trauma are ineffective.

Yet, in spite of all the signs pointing to a traumatized population, the fifth edition of the *Diagnostic and Statistical Manual of Mental Disorders* (commonly known as *DSM-5*), published by the American Psychiatric Association, defines trauma (within the context of PTSD) as exposure to actual or threatened death, serious injury, or sexual violence. That's the extent the governing body of psychiatric conditions defines trauma. The implication is that if you are experiencing PTSD that doesn't fit into any of those criteria, then you are in fact not traumatized. This is both an insulting and archaic overture to the millions who are experiencing deep and traumatic suffering at the hands of countless events, issues, threats, and victimization.

I'm reminded of the great comedian George Carlin when I think about the origins of PTSD in American culture. For years, part of his monologue included a bit on the etymology of the clinical term "post-traumatic stress disorder." After World War I, we simply referred to it as "shell shock," which then morphed into "battle fatigue," and then it finally landed at what we now call PTSD. The linguistics, while meant to be funny in Carlin's bit, emphasize that we really don't know much about trauma at all. The mere acknowledgement that it even exists only dates back to the mid-twentieth century.

When it comes to treating it, we are in the infancy of even being able to provide options to patients that are remotely effective. Talk therapy, exposure therapy, support groups, psychiatric medications, and even more modern therapeutic approaches like eye movement desensitization and reprocessing (EMDR) are essentially shots in the dark. Efficacy rates are low and often inaccurate, probably due to the fact that there is no one method we can turn to for effective data.

It's all put into a blender, and the end result is a tapestry of unreliable insight into what's working and what isn't.

Trauma's Wide Reach

Fortunately, many modern psychologists, like Dr. Gabor Maté, have widened the lens for how trauma occurs and thus have affected many more people than we know. Maté's theory centers on several key principles: early life experiences, the impact of adverse childhood experiences (ACEs), the biological and psychological effects of trauma, and the importance of compassion and healing. Maté emphasizes the critical role of early life experiences, especially in childhood, in shaping an individual's neurological, psychological, and emotional development. Traumatic events or adverse experiences during this formative period can have profound and long-lasting effects on an individual's health and behavior. The problem with many of those events is that they become repressed memories, and uncovering them is oftentimes scary. As we will later discuss, this is a perfect example of why certain psychedelics can aid in uncovering these traumas without fear.

ACEs include various forms of trauma such as abuse, neglect, family dysfunction, and household challenges, like substance abuse or mental illness. Maté underscores the correlation between ACEs and a higher risk of physical and mental health issues later in life, including addiction, chronic diseases, mental health disorders, and difficulties in forming healthy relationships. What we are imprinted with at an early age can affect us negatively in our adult lives. Those imprints matter and become the blueprints for how we see the world. Maté also delves into the physiological and psychological mechanisms through which trauma affects the body and mind. Chronic stress resulting from early trauma can disrupt the body's stress response systems, impacting brain development, hormonal regulation, and immune function. This dysregulation can contribute to various health conditions and psychological struggles.

Maté advocates for a compassionate approach to individuals impacted by trauma. He emphasizes the importance of providing a nurturing environment, empathetic support, and opportunities for healing and recovery to break the cycle of trauma and its potential intergenerational transmission. Breaking the cycle is one of the most challenging elements in healthy family development. "Hurt people, hurt people" has become a cliché, and for good reason. Without the proper education for how trauma manifests in our lives, it's far too easy to pass it on to others.

By focusing on highlighting the profound and pervasive impact of traumatic early life experiences on human health and well-being, his theory encourages those of us who are suffering to get more in touch with the past by viewing it as not something to be afraid of and instead as part of the story that has shaped us. By recognizing the role of trauma in shaping individuals' lives, understanding its far-reaching effects, and emphasizing the importance of compassion, understanding, and holistic approaches to healing that address both the biological and psychological dimensions of trauma, we can better understand how trauma is affecting far more people than we thought and hopefully find a better way forward in treating it.

From my experience as someone who has experienced high levels of trauma in my active substance abuse addiction and bearing witness to so many seeking relief from PTSD in the psychedelic space, my main takeaway is that it's not a contest. None of us should ever be prone to label one person's suffering as being more severe than someone else's. Of course there is a big difference between the pain that a rape victim sustains compared to a lesser impact source of trauma, but my point is that we must encourage all healers, both medical and otherwise, to increase their level of compassion and acceptance to anyone who is experiencing traumatic pain. Your worst day is just as valid as anyone else's worst day, and it deserves to be looked at with compassion.

Working with Suffering

The Buddha was wise to ponder the essence of the human condition and determine that before enlightenment is to happen, we all must observe and acknowledge that suffering is a core element in holding back growth. He did not simply say, "Find God and you will be free of suffering," or suggest that there was some magic path that shortcut our road to wellness. Rather, he suggested a psycho-spiritual method that encourages us to take a contemplative look at where we are rooted in suffering.

The Buddhist philosophy on suffering is known as "Dukkha" in the ancient language of Pali. Dukkha encompasses various forms of unsatisfactoriness, suffering, or dissatisfaction that are inherent in human existence. Understanding and transcending suffering is a key aspect of the Four Noble Truths, a fundamental doctrine of Buddhism—in fact it's made clear in the first one. The first Noble Truth highlights that Dukkha is an inevitable aspect of existence, affecting everyone regardless of age, social status, or circumstance. Whether it's physical pain, mental anguish, the fleeting nature of joy, or the inability to find lasting satisfaction in material possessions or achievements, Dukkha is seen as a universal human experience. As far as I can make out, that simple philosophy applies to everyone, and if we all have the courage to look within, we will find that some form of it exists in our lives.

Buddhist teachings do not deny the existence of happiness or joy in life but rather highlight that even pleasurable experiences are transient and subject to change. The emphasis lies in understanding the impermanent, unsatisfactory nature of all conditioned phenomena and finding liberation from the cycle of suffering through spiritual practice and insight. Buddhism, as it turns out, paints a wonderful parallel picture for how psychedelics can be so useful for treating trauma. Suffering, when unacknowledged, can turn to trauma, and trauma, when untreated, can block any sense of joy or happiness in one's life. The traumatic residue can get so severe that even the good parts of one's life feel empty.

The world is at a crisis point right now, and the sooner we acknowledge the level of suffering all around and approach healing in new ways, the sooner we can move toward global and collective solutions.

MDMA and PTSD Relief

Psychedelic-assisted therapy for the treatment of PTSD looks like it has the potential to not only revolutionize healing for populations that have been largely ignored (e.g., vets, first responders, sexual abuse survivors, and countless others) but also expand how we define suffering, pain, and the origins of trauma.

I've always been a little gun shy when proclaiming that any psychedelic is a miracle cure for anything. There are always those who it doesn't work for, and blind zealotry never works well for any cause. But I do admit that if there's ever been a treatment that is so perfectly suited for the treatment of PTSD, it is MDMA. Its success (so far) in the treatment of PTSD is almost hard to believe. The effectiveness that MDMA has had in treating PTSD is reflected in the published efficacy rates from the Phase 2 clinical trials (which have led to Phase 3) sponsored by MAPS. They reported that approximately 61 to 68 percent of participants no longer met the criteria for PTSD diagnosis after undergoing MDMA-assisted therapy. This was compared to about 25 to 30 percent of participants in the control group (which received a placebo or standard therapy) who no longer met the PTSD diagnosis criteria.

It's very important to outline how this therapy works and why it is so effective. The participants in the clinical trials are not just given the drug in the hopes that it will lessen the PTSD symptoms on its own. They are given three medicine sessions that are preceded by intensive prep work, integration sessions in between, and follow-up therapy afterward—all of which are done by a clinically trained psychotherapist. It's the combination of the drug's miraculous knack for opening up the heart and increasing empathy with a trained professional who can help piece together the client's issues in a way that is both compassionate and constructive.

I point this out because there are a great number of people who are suffering from PTSD who have not been able to qualify for legal clinical trial participation and are seeking this treatment. Even if they do find a qualified person to take them through this process, legally or otherwise, it's vital to remember that the MDMA journeys are just one part of the process and won't do all the work for them. They must be willing to engage in the multi-tiered process of therapy, MDMA, a strong support system, and an overall willingness to talk about their issues. The way the drug works on the brain, however, is completely unique and puts into question why exactly this compound is so effective at treating trauma.

PTSD, when left untreated, changes people's brains. It can increase activity in the amygdala, where fear is regulated and processed, and reduce activity in the prefrontal cortex, where rational decision-making takes place. This is why it can become so difficult to make sound decisions when trauma is activated, and instead violence, drug use, or dissociation may occur. MDMA does the opposite, decreasing activity in the amygdala and increasing activity in the prefrontal cortex. MDMA also stimulates the release of the hormones prolactin and oxytocin, which are associated with bonding, affiliation, and love, facilitating the therapeutic alliance between patient and therapist and increasing the effectiveness of psychotherapy. MDMA also stimulates the release of the neurotransmitters serotonin, dopamine, and norepinephrine, producing a complex symphony of effects that help the drug enhance the benefits of psychotherapy.

How MDMA works on the brain and why it is so effective in the treatment of PTSD can be broken down into a few categories of understanding:

- **Enhanced therapeutic alliance:** MDMA, when administered in a therapeutic setting, promotes a state of increased trust, empathy, and emotional openness. This can significantly enhance the therapeutic alliance between the patient and therapist, allowing individuals with PTSD to engage more comfortably in the therapeutic process.

- **Reduction of fear and anxiety:** MDMA's pharmacological effects include reducing fear and anxiety responses while increasing feelings of safety and trust. This can be especially beneficial for individuals with PTSD, as it allows them to approach traumatic memories or experiences without overwhelming fear and resistance. When on the medicine, MDMA temporarily alters the amygdala's governance of fear and increases the participant's willingness to talk about those fears.

- **Facilitated emotional processing:** MDMA can facilitate emotional processing by lowering defenses and inhibitions. This can enable individuals to explore and process traumatic memories or emotions in a more adaptive and less distressing manner during therapy sessions.

- **Promotion of empathy and compassion:** The empathogenic effects of MDMA, such as increased feelings of empathy and compassion, can help individuals with PTSD develop a compassionate and nonjudgmental perspective toward themselves and their traumatic experiences.

- **Neurobiological effects:** MDMA has been shown to modulate certain brain areas and neurotransmitter systems involved in emotional regulation and memory processing. It may assist in reconsolidating traumatic memories in a less emotionally distressing way.

This provides some insight into how and why empathogens work and how they open up our hearts and allow us to communicate parts of ourselves that are normally difficult to talk about. What I find most amazing and even counterintuitive is that MDMA allows many participants to look at their trauma with a newfound sense of compassion, forgiveness, and love. I can attest to the fact that in my normal waking state, when I am engaged in traditional therapeutic methods like talk therapy, I am not quick to associate my trauma with compassion or forgiveness. The default position of anger and confusion have always contributed to me making very slow progress in my own healing.

The greatest miracle I've seen is when I hear the stories from veterans who have found some relief through MDMA therapy. Jonathan Lubecky, who now serves as the Veterans and Governmental Affairs Liaison for the Multidisciplinary Association for Psychedelic Studies' Public Benefit Corporation (MAPS PBC), was in the Marines and Army and was active duty in Iraq from 2005 to 2006. In recounting his story with The American Legion's TBI/PTSD Suicide Prevention Committee, he said, "Within two months of coming back from Iraq, I went to a bar to have a few drinks for Christmas Eve. I heard church bells and realized I should have been [at the hospital]. I went there. They were full and told me to go away."

He went to various hospitals and doctors and didn't get the help he needed. He continued, "I was given six Xanax and told not to take them all at the same time. They asked if I had firearms at home. I said yes. They said I needed to go home at three o'clock on Christmas morning and give my firearms to my neighbor, waking them up, and then to come back after the holiday. After five (suicide) attempts, hospitalizations, everything, I had an intern slide a piece of paper across the desk and say, 'Don't open this until you leave. I'm not supposed to tell you about it.' It said, 'Google MDMA PTSD,'" Lubecky said. "I discovered MAPS was doing a clinical trial. Because two people had dropped out before completing the full trial because they felt healed after one or two sessions, there was enough room for me."

Lubecky took his first dose of MDMA in November 2014. "In 2022 I was healed of PTSD," he said. "There are not many people on this planet who can say that. One of the biggest lies we were ever told was that PTSD is a permanent condition. Whether it's

MDMA-assisted therapies, regular talk therapies, or other therapies, I am proof that PTSD can be eliminated."

Jonathan's story is just one of many that have not only changed how we approach treating trauma but also how we think of psychedelics in general. The impact veterans have created in sharing their MDMA journeys has been one of the great cultural shifts in how society and more establishment-based naysayers are now talking about psychedelics. The stories combined with the data have changed the minds of people I never thought could be changed.

Veterans are a population that, no matter what side of the political fence you are on, are people we support and want the best for. It's become a bipartisan issue to call out Veterans Affairs and their lack of effectiveness in treating our vets when they come home from war. That reality is not something that too many politicians, liberal or conservative, disagree on. According to the VA, on average 16.8 veterans died by suicide per day in 2021. This number has been pretty consistent since the VA started tracking veteran suicides in 2001. These numbers are not something that anyone can or should ignore.

Soon after Rick Doblin started MAPS in 1986, he said that its mission would be rooted in making MDMA a legal treatment for veterans with PTSD, and he has since found success not only in the treatments but in how MAPS's work has shifted public opinion. Doblin wrote in an article published by centrist *Time Magazine*, "US and global drug prohibition has for decades delayed medical research into the healing properties of Schedule 1 drugs. Now that this research is finally being conducted, we're learning that enormous suffering and many suicides could have been prevented over these decades. It's long past time for the mainstreaming of the medical use of psychedelics and marijuana, and for replacing prohibition and criminalization with public health approaches to reducing drug abuse. In a post-prohibition world, we'll finally recognize that."

So, it's become a wonderful synchronicity that the treatment of one population (vets) can now open the door for others suffering. Psychedelics have long held promise to treat a myriad of conditions, but the War on Drugs and the unwritten culture war against drug users have gotten in the way of being able to make any real progress. Sometimes all the positive data and research isn't enough. Sometimes it takes a certain group of people to penetrate the hearts and minds of the opposition. Stories that are rooted in grounded and compassionate transformation and are far removed from radical counterculture claims of psychedelic mysticism are sometimes what we need.

Other Psychedelics and PTSD Relief

The psychedelic influence in treating veteran trauma isn't only limited to MDMA. MAPS has also sponsored a study in treating PTSD in vets with the self-administered use of cannabis, and a wonderful film called *Soldiers of the Vine* details the journey of six American veterans who go to Peru to participate in a ten-day Ayahuasca ritual to treat their PTSD.

Ian Benouis, a veteran and plant medicine activist who brought the group to Peru said of his own healing and journey to helping others, "Well, I did my military service and got out. I was a Blackhawk helicopter pilot during Operation Just Cause in Panama right before Iraq and Afghanistan, and drank Ayahuasca three more times without really knowing I was healing myself. It wasn't until a couple of years ago when I reconnected with veterans at a conference on veterans and cannabis, and they started telling their stories [that I realized I had been undergoing a healing process via psychedelics]. I already knew there were issues with PTSD, cocktails of pharmaceuticals that didn't work for lots of people, and of course the suicides, but when they started telling their stories, it was like a psychedelic to me, a medicine, and I started crying. I was purging up all this stuff, and was like, 'Why is this happening to me? I don't have war traumas.' That started round 2.0 of my healing. I realized what psychedelics had done for me, and how that healing had gotten me to where I could raise a family and be a good husband and father. And now to complete my healing, I could return to the medicine and share it with others."

Because of all these stories contributing to the changing narrative around psychedelics, a few bipartisan members of Congress have added psychedelic healing to a major defense spending bill. The bill's psychedelic sections require the Department of Defense to facilitate access for military veterans for the treatment of PTSD or traumatic brain injury (TBI). The provisions allow for participation in studies that use psilocybin, MDMA, ibogaine, and 5-MeO DMT.

Psychedelics and Personal Trauma Relief

In conclusion, I want to share a personal story of someone I worked with in the psychedelic space. I reached out to several subsets of these people so they could share their stories on trauma. The following story is from a "first timer," a woman over the age of fifty who had a lifelong history of depression that had its roots in childhood trauma. What she took away from her psilocybin journey was a very revealing look into what she was not able to recognize prior.

"Eating the mushrooms was easy. They didn't taste like much. Very dry but easy to get down. But I did immediately feel like I was doing something special. Something that would give me insight into what I've been holding back. I laid back and did some long slow breaths as I waited for the medicine to kick in, and sure enough after what felt like forever, they took ahold of me. It was sudden and powerful. I was scared. I'm glad that I had a guide there to remind me that I was safe and loved and one that helped me to breathe through these changes. Most of what occurred was not part of the plan I laid out going into the session. The medicine, I was told, has its own agenda. That also scared me. Once I surrendered to it and got comfortable in this altered space, my fifty-plus years of being a traumatized woman became clear. The roots of the trauma were foggy and mixed, but how I behaved in the world was crystal clear. The tone of voice that I use in conflict with my husband and children was appearing in my ears, booming like a church bell. Over and over again, I could hear this subtle thing that I do. This subtle way of talking to my loved ones that wasn't love at all. It was scornful and judgmental. So loud.

That realization made me sad and reminded me of the person I didn't want to be in the world. I was taking my trauma out on others. This went on for what felt like hours, but I later found out it was only about an hour. I asked my guide how to forgive myself. I then started to hear that voice getting dimmer and dimmer, and my body felt at ease and even pleasurable. When it was all over, I wanted nothing more than to not be that person that I had been. I wanted to love my family the way that they should be loved and to not let my trauma dictate my waking reality. It's a process but this one session lit the fire of that process."

I never thought I'd see a day where so many people outside of the traditional psychedelic communities are able to share a newfound acceptance for these magical compounds, including their use in treating trauma. It's a brave new world full of compelling data, moving personal stories, and changing minds around these new healing methods. I'm confident that the next ten years will uncover even more revelatory shifts in how we heal with psychedelics and how they continue to change our understanding of trauma.

5

Cognitive Liberty

Why Thinking for Yourself Still Matters

"Think for yourself and question authority."

—Timothy Leary

Cognitive liberty in my view is at the forefront of what it means to evolve within our own lifetime. The post-industrial age and what it has done to limit the path of self-inquiry and all-around growth is very noticeable if you look around. We are encouraged, if not mandated, to conform to the K–12 model of education and then mold ourselves into a career that provides advancement and promotes conformity. As a society we aren't encouraged to break against the stream of normality by diving deeper into questioning the very nature of reality. To question the systemic shackles of society is to be labeled an outlaw—god forbid too many of us start thinking for ourselves!

Cognitive liberty encompasses the rights and freedoms pertaining to one's own consciousness, thoughts, and cognitive processes, and is integral to individual autonomy and self-determination. In some respect, this language alone was rare for the average man to speak of prior to the '60s, even though these ideas were enshrined into our founding documents like the Bill of Rights. But in practice, the puritanical roots of American life have always stifled those who think against the grain. I believe philosophers like Ralph Waldo Emerson and Henry David Thoreau replanted the seeds that encouraged the individual to go within and discover what it means to explore our inner worlds.

Cognitive liberty also encapsulates the right to freely explore, alter, and choose one's mental states without undue interference or coercion. This liberty manifests in various forms, each crucial in shaping our understanding of personal autonomy and the boundaries of cognitive sovereignty.

At its core, cognitive liberty includes the freedom to think, believe, and express oneself without censorship or repression. It embodies the right to hold diverse opinions, engage in critical thinking, and freely articulate thoughts and ideas without fear of persecution or suppression by authorities or societal norms. Our ancestors knew this, and from what we've uncovered through archeology and early written history, we can see that many ancient cultures used psychedelics as a tool for disruption.

Ethnobotanist and ethnomycologist Giorgio Samorini studied the use of psychoactive substances for more than twenty years, conducting research in Africa, Latin America, India, and Europe. Upon encountering the 10,000-year-old cave paintings in Tassili, Algeria, he described it in his writing as, "a series of masked figures in line and hieratically dressed or dressed as dancers surrounded by long and lively festoons of geometrical designs of different kinds." Each dancer "holds a mushroom-like object in the right hand," but the key visual depiction are the lines that "come out of this object to reach the central part of the head of the dancer." These "could signify an indirect association or non-material fluid passing from the object held in the right hand and the mind." An interpretation of this metaphor most likely points to "the universal mental value induced by hallucinogenic mushrooms and vegetals, which is often of a mystical and spiritual nature."

In Terence McKenna's *Food of the Gods*, he writes about the same cave paintings saying, "The shamans are dancing with fists full of mushrooms and also have mushrooms sprouting out of their bodies. In one instance they are shown running joyfully, surrounded by the geometric structures of their hallucinations. The pictorial evidence seems incontrovertible."

What were these ancient Algerians doing 10,000 years ago? Clearly it was important enough to them that they memorialized it in art so it would serve to document their mushroom-fueled celebration of the mysteries of life. Do you think the people depicted in these ancient cave paintings placed any sort of morality around the use of the mushroom? Did they argue about whether or not it was right or wrong to explore their consciousness with these tools? We can't be sure since there is very little written history of the era, but what we can assume is that our ancestors were cognitive libertarians at heart.

The Eleusinian Mysteries of ancient Greece also date back thousands of years and are considered to be one of ancient Greece's most revered and secret celebrations. The rituals themselves were void of the class and gender restrictions of the time and seemed to have no hierarchy at all. Slaves and women could participate alongside some of the more well-known attendants, like Socrates and Aristotle. The festival started in early September in Eleusis, a town fourteen miles from Athens, and was known as the most mysterious of the ancient Greek world. The major multiday rites of the Mysteries were closely related to the myth of Demeter and her daughter Persephone. The sacred story of their bitter separation and joyful reunion served as catalysts for the spiritual enlightenment of the initiates, and the rituals were intended to evoke an overwhelming and ineffable experience. The initiates would sip a drink known as kykeon, a psychedelic intoxicant whose exact formula is unknown, but evidence suggests it contained a form of ergot—the natural world's precursor to LSD.

By all accounts, the festival went on for nine days under starry skies with lit torches, music, and celebration that, all together, induced a sort of ritualistic chaos. Each day would gradually take them to another level of realizations that got to the very core of the expanding philosophy of the day. Socrates proclaimed that "excellence and virtue" was rooted within and should spill outward from the righteous individual. And Pausanias included ideas like living piously, honoring parents, and glorifying gods. Cultural and behavioral change were emitted from the festival attendees and went on to form so much of the core ancient philosophical tenets of Ancient Greece.

As discussed earlier, the Aztecs, one of the most well-known and fascinating ancient Mesoamerican civilizations that thrived in present-day Mexico, had a rich cultural tapestry interwoven with spiritual practices and rituals. Among their various traditions, the Aztecs' use of psychedelic mushrooms stands out as a significant aspect of their religious ceremonies, cultural beliefs, and understanding of altered states of consciousness.

Central to the Aztec society was their reverence for nature and the cosmos. You can see that deep appreciation depicted in Aztec art and symbology. They attributed spiritual significance to various natural elements, including plants and fungi. By that I mean they had a deep respect for plants as teachers. One such teacher was the fungus *Psilocybe mexicana*, colloquially known as "teonanácatl" or "flesh of the gods." This particular species of psychedelic mushroom contained the psychoactive compounds psilocybin and psilocin, but we can't be sure how much. We are sure that they induced altered states of perception, vivid hallucinations, and profound spiritual experiences when used in the ritualized manner of their culture.

Historical accounts and archaeological evidence suggest that the Aztecs, alongside other Indigenous Mesoamerican cultures, integrated psychedelic mushrooms into their religious ceremonies and rituals. The use of these mushrooms was far from a recreational model and was deeply rooted in their spiritual practices and understanding of the divine. This was serious work to them, not play. This was also the embodiment of a culture living by the idea that by allowing citizens to change their consciousness with the aid of plant medicines could make for a better world and a better understanding of what it means to live in harmony. The "flesh of the gods" was believed to connect individuals with the spirit world, facilitating communication with deities, ancestors, and other supernatural entities. Revered spiritual leaders with profound knowledge of these substances would ingest mushrooms as a means to enter altered states of consciousness. Through these states, they sought visions, guidance, and healing powers to aid their communities.

The importance that Aztecs placed on these rituals is shown in where they held them. They often occurred in elaborate ceremonial centers such as the Templo Mayor in the capital city of Tenochtitlan. During regular religious festivals and ceremonies, the sacred mushrooms were consumed alongside other offerings to honor gods like Xochipilli, the Aztec deity of flowers, love, and psychoactive plants. Beyond their quest for divine bliss and sacred understanding of the world, the Aztecs' utilization of psychedelic mushrooms extended into medicinal practices as well. They believed psilocybin to possess healing properties and used them to treat various ailments, both physical and psychological. Sadly, many of their homeopathic recipes were lost to time.

Despite the cultural significance and spiritual reverence attached to these mushrooms, their use declined following the Spanish conquest of the Aztec Empire in the sixteenth century. The Spanish colonizers viewed Indigenous rituals, including the consumption of psychedelic mushrooms, as pagan and blasphemous, leading to the suppression and prohibition of these practices. This is an example of the reason why ancient mystical rituals that included psychedelics went dormant for many years: Christian-based colonialism was an enemy to Indigenous culture and rituals that the colonizers could not understand. Fortunately, the resurgence of interest in the cultural and Indigenous practices of cultures like the Aztecs has sparked a renewed sense of their profound cultural significance that continues to intrigue and inspire curiosity in our modern world.

Ancient Algeria, Greece, and Mexico are just three of numerous examples of how and where ancient psychedelic rituals took place. I chose these three brief explorations because they dot various corners of the globe ranging from Europe to Africa to Latin America. Somewhere down the line, most of us have an ancient relative who used psychedelics as a ritualized gateway for understanding the universe and their own mind and getting closer to God. Inside your DNA is a built-in quest to dive deeper into the understanding of consciousness, spirit, and the universe around you with the aid of the natural world's wonders, including psychedelic plants and vegetables. This was not a controversial opinion for millennia. In fact, it was a de facto standard in the understanding of evolution.

So, what happened? Where did the deep acceptance and practice of exploring our consciousness with the aid of psychedelics go? Why did cognitive liberty become such a hotly debated fundamental right? Why did the right to change our consciousness as we see fit like the ancient Greeks and Aztecs get relegated to merely being a primitive example of tribal living by European colonialists?

The Disappearance of Psychedelic Traditions in Many Cultures

We know from a historical perspective that the ancient use of psychedelic drugs was deeply embedded in the cultural, spiritual, and medicinal practices of many civilizations across the globe. This is not debated. However, the disappearance of these practices from modern society can be attributed to several interconnected factors spanning social, political, religious, and scientific realms. I've suggested six areas here that have taken us further away from the practice of using plant medicines to change the way we think and see. Modernization comes with many benefits, but it also has many pitfalls.

- **Colonization and cultural suppression:** The arrival of European colonizers in various parts of the world led to the suppression and eradication of Indigenous cultural practices, including the use of psychedelic substances. Conquest and colonization often involved the imposition of new religious beliefs and the prohibition of Indigenous rituals deemed pagan or sacrilegious by the colonizers. Colonists tended to view the people they were colonizing in a xenophobic light. Rather than learn from them, they persecuted them—even the wise elders of the lands they were conquering. These colonists came to a land for the bounties it contained but then also forced their way of thinking onto it.

- **Religious and moral stigmatization:** As societies transitioned toward organized religions with stringent moral codes, the use of psychedelic drugs was increasingly demonized and condemned. Many religious authorities deemed altered states of consciousness induced by these substances as heretical or sinful, contributing to their suppression. Why is that? The answer is simple: if you take psychedelics and form your own view of God that contradicts the written dogma, then you become a threat. The post-Crusade world left no room for others to worship in ways that were unusual or different.

- **Legal restrictions and prohibition:** Governments and authorities, influenced by social attitudes and moral perceptions rooted in colonialist belief systems, enacted laws to criminalize the possession and use of psychedelic drugs. The War on Drugs, which led to strict legal prohibitions categorizing possession of these substances as illegal and punishable offenses, is simply a war on people the government doesn't like. Each iteration of it demonizes specific racial, ethnic, and class segments of our population. What better way to persecute them than demonize their behaviors?

- **Lack of scientific understanding:** With the advancement of modern science, there emerged a knowledge gap regarding psychedelic substances between the ancient cultural wisdom and scientific understanding. These drugs were often misunderstood and classified as harmful without comprehensive research into their potential benefits. What we now refer to as the "Scientific Method" dismisses any knowledge from the ancient world or lived experience. We see this same symptomatic discrimination in areas like naturopathy versus pharmaceuticals or holistic treatments versus psychiatry.

- **Shift in societal values:** As societies evolved and industrialized, there was a shift toward a more materialistic and productivity-focused lifestyle. This shift in values diminished the importance placed on spiritual exploration, communal rituals, and traditional healing practices involving psychedelic substances. The industrial revolution changed the nature of man, turning them into a worker as opposed to a thinker or philosopher.

- **Loss of knowledge of Indigenous traditions:** The suppression of Indigenous cultures, combined with the passing of generations and the lack of transmission of traditional knowledge, resulted in the loss or fragmentation of ancient practices involving psychedelic drugs. This loss of cultural heritage contributed to these rituals fading from modern society. Curanderas in Mexico and Native American healers all suffered the same fate. Their destruction led to their rituals being forgotten and becoming an almost folklorish tale of what once was, not what is.

Luckily, within the modern psychedelic renaissance, there has been a resurgence of interest in how ancient and Indigenous cultures used psychedelic substances. How they sat around the fire, told stories, and worshipped is interwoven into the use of psychedelics, and there is a newfound sense of interest in and respect for those rituals.

The disappearance of widespread ancient practices involving psychedelic drugs is a complex interplay of historical, cultural, religious, and legal factors that an entire book could be written about. While these substances have largely been sidelined, there is a growing movement to revisit and integrate ancient wisdom with contemporary scientific knowledge to explore the therapeutic and spiritual dimensions of these substances in a responsible and informed manner.

Cognitive Liberty and Psychedelics

For obvious reasons, one facet of cognitive liberty that I am incredibly passionate about—and often what I mean when discussing the proliferation of psychedelics—is the exploration of altered states of consciousness. This form of exploration allows individuals to delve into profound introspection, spiritual experiences, and expanded consciousness, fostering personal growth and self-discovery. The modern medicalization movement's focus on mental health has distanced itself from this theme, and I think it's time it was brought back into the forefront as a core principle for why psychedelics should be understood and considered.

Most religious and spiritual practices involve altering consciousness through meditation, rituals, or ceremonies, aiming to achieve transcendental experiences or deeper connections with the self and the universe. Even the major religions of today have a sect or element that believes this. Cognitive liberty encompasses the right to engage in such practices without external interference or restriction. Therefore, why our society says it's okay to do one but not the other should be talked about as the hypocrisy that it is.

However, the placement of cognitive liberty as a human right (which I maintain to be true) still intersects with ethical, legal, and societal considerations that some say threatens a "civilized" society. Balancing personal freedom with potential risks to oneself and others, addressing societal perceptions, and navigating regulatory frameworks remain significant challenges. Still, I choose to trust people. I believe that with proper education and the rejection of false narratives around the safe use of psychedelics, we can proclaim our fundamental right to change our way of looking at the world. Our ancient forefathers and foremothers believed this then, so why shouldn't we today? I believe the navigation of regulations and the dissemination of safe use protocols are only obstacles and not deal breakers.

Cognitive liberty represents the inherent right of individuals to govern their own mental landscapes, explore diverse states of consciousness, and make choices concerning their cognitive well-being. It encompasses a spectrum of freedoms, from the right to altered states of consciousness to the autonomy of mental privacy. It is a multifaceted endeavor that requires nuanced consideration of ethical, legal, and societal implications while respecting individual autonomy and the diversity of human experiences. Why is this so important though? When stripping ourselves away from the vast and effective mental health benefits that psychedelics can offer, why is it so important that we carve out a right to explore our own consciousness and minds as we see fit?

Cognitive Spontaneity

What does it mean to explore our minds, souls, and cognitive framework in this manner? The answer varies between each person who has used psychedelic drugs for this purpose. Each person would give a different answer and a unique framework for what was revealed in the exploration of their own extraordinary minds. I find it useful to begin with the observations of thoughts and what that process looks like.

If one is to sit quietly and observe their thoughts, they will notice a nonlinear and seemingly random way in which their thoughts dance around their mind and then make themselves known to the observer. If you were able to write down every single thought as it appeared in the silent void, it would resemble the diary of a madman. Our brain is firing on so many concurrent instances of perception that it becomes nearly impossible to recognize them all at once. This is why speech and word choice are very useful ways of extracting the thoughts that are most relevant to us at any given moment. This is also why meditation is so challenging at first. There are simply too many thoughts to quiet the mind and focus it on our breath. Buddhists call it the "monkey mind," the "unsettled, restless, capricious, whimsical, fanciful, inconstant, confused, indecisive, uncontrollable" thoughts we experience in our minds.

The "monkey mind" draws an analogy between the mind's behavior and that of a restless monkey, leaping from branch to branch without pause or focus. I've spent a lot of time in Vrindavan, India, a holy town that may have as many monkeys as it does people. The monkeys, for that particular reason, have become so accustomed to the human population that they don't hesitate for a moment if they need to grab food from your hands when they are hungry or snatch the glasses off your face simply to amuse themselves. My time there really helped me fully understand what the Buddhists meant when coming up with this metaphor. Unhinged, restless, desperate, and unpredictable. Are we talking about our mind or the monkeys? One can't be sure.

Without attention to this state of being, it often leads to feelings of agitation, anxiety, and an inability to concentrate or find inner peace. Tried-and-true methods like meditation, yoga, and pranayama (breathwork) are very effective in helping to slow the entire process down. They don't erase it, but they can be successful in getting the observer to view one sequence of thoughts at a time rather than get completely overwhelmed by the sheer volume of activity that takes up space in their mind.

By cultivating awareness and practicing mindfulness, individuals can observe the fluctuations of the mind without getting entangled in its constant stream of thoughts. This practice allows one to develop a sense of inner calmness, detach from the restless tendencies of the mind, and gain better control over the monkey mind, leading to increased clarity, focus, and a deeper understanding of the self.

The concept of the monkey mind serves as a reminder of the need for mental discipline and the cultivation of a daily mindfulness practice to overcome distractions and anxiety and make peace with the constant influx of stories that our minds create.

Psychedelics and the Monkey Mind

What I'm about to say next often scares psychedelic first timers. Being on psychedelics can, at first, feel like the opposite of meditation: a million streams of awareness are all appearing at once, sometimes seeming like a chaotic download of every possible option happening simultaneously. It can be overwhelming to experience your mind's waking state in overdrive—to feel that sense of cognitive enhancement that reenacts every memory, event, or idea you've ever had. On one hand, you may feel an overwhelming sense of being alive and the realization that you're much smarter than you've led yourself to believe, and on the other, you may feel a state of chaos and disorder that has no end in sight.

This is until one surrenders into the beautiful void of streamed consciousness that then transitions into one fantastically peaceful feeling of tuning into "the one." There are many variations of "the one" in my opinion. Ram Dass meant it as the one singular stream of unconditional love that we call God, and others may refer to it as the perfection of all things in the universe. These are both true. I also see it as the experience of tuning into one stream of infinite consciousness, which includes your thoughts as well as the endless energetic influence of every other thought that has ever occurred. I find myself coming up with ideas during a psychedelic session that I never dreamed I was capable of having. In fact, Ram Dass once said of the LSD experience, "LSD is a catalyst or a tool for accessing deep parts of the psyche that are usually not available to us."

It's profoundly different from sober consciousness. The effects can vary widely depending on the specific substance, dosage, set (voyager's mindset), setting, and individual intentions. However, several general patterns often emerge. In my experience, I have now become so familiar with the patterns that they no longer overwhelm me, even though they can still surprise me.

Entheogens tend to intensify and amplify thoughts, emotions, and sensory experiences. Colors become vibrant, and music becomes a multilayered tapestry of sound and vision. When things go well, this leads to deep introspection, heightened creativity, and an enhanced awareness of one's feelings and their place in the world. Especially poignant are autobiographical recollections that cause you to take a look at your life from every perspective other than the one you normally see it through. Psychedelics alter the usual patterns of thinking, leading to a nonlinear or nonsequential thought process. Ideas may seem to flow more freely, and associations between seemingly unrelated concepts can become more apparent. This can result in a more expansive and open-minded perspective, allowing for novel connections and insights. Think of this like an orgasmic flow of emotional and cognitive synesthesia, where you connect ideas that you previously thought could not be connected.

I believe the spontaneity that occurs is at the hands of the medicine coupled with your ability to surrender to it. You're not steering the ship. It's up to you to surrender and receive what's being shown, not to force a certain outcome that your ego wants to happen. This is why many who go deep in the psychedelic space report a dissolution of the ego—the sense of individual self—while on psychedelics. This can lead to a feeling of interconnectedness with others, nature, or the universe. Psychedelics also challenge your sense of everyday ego, challenging your notions of when you think you're right. When you realize you're not as right as you think you are and you don't know as much as you think you know, there is a tremendous sense of relief. I find it reassuring to know that, even in my middle-age years, there is still so much to learn about myself and the world around me.

Thoughts might encompass a sense of unity and transcendental experiences that go beyond conventional boundaries of self. This emotional amplification can lead to profound introspection, cathartic releases, or, in some cases, increased vulnerability and sensitivity. "Starving, naked, and afraid" as Ginsberg said in "Howl."

Despite the intensified mental activity and newfound sense of rebirth, people also often report an increased sense of mindfulness and being in the present moment. Knowing how you work and how your mind operates when it is free from the restrictions of ego and the noose of the stories we tell ourselves over and over again is freedom at the ultimate level. Our ancestors knew this and were steadfast in their adoption of cognitive liberty as a sacred birthright. Entire societies and cultures were built around the desire to "know thyself" and, by doing so, become more in tune with the tribe around us. No matter where you find yourself in today's world, I'm sure most of us could agree that striving for that, even in the twenty-first century, is a good idea.

6

Magic and Mysticism

The Hero's Journey

"Whole systems of underground life beneath 'consciousness of the ordinary field.' He says: 'we cannot, I think, avoid the conclusion that in religion we have a department of human nature with unusually close relations to the trans-marginal or subliminal region.'"

—William James

In my early days of psychedelic exploration, ages fifteen to twenty-five, people in my circle were not aware of any research studies or clinical trials that said using psychedelic drugs could help treat depression, anxiety, or lessen the effects of PTSD. Our only mission when using psychedelics was to explore our minds, the nature of reality, and, if we were lucky, get closer to God.

That was really our only intention: to go with God.

Alan Watts, the brilliant philosopher and interpreter of Eastern philosophy, gave lectures on public radio on Sunday nights when I was growing up. I would tape them and pore over them like I found a map to a lost treasure that would reveal something big. What that was, I wasn't entirely sure, but I knew it was important.

Watts said, "The mystical experience is ordinarily called cosmic consciousness, unitary consciousness, or a sense of oneness with the universe. And this is, of course, the psychological basis of religion. But the interesting thing is that it's beginning to be possible to produce this experience with chemicals, such as LSD, and indeed certain other chemicals . . . But you can't have the experience unless you are prepared to see God in all His forms, all His manifestations, or Her forms or Her manifestations, and everything that exists. If you are unwilling to see that, you can't have the experience."

This reflects Watts's perspective on how psychedelics, particularly LSD, can induce states of consciousness akin to mystical experiences. However, he emphasizes that such experiences are contingent upon one's openness to perceiving the interconnectedness and divinity in all aspects of existence. These were the seeds that for me were the primary motivations for wanting to use psychedelics. And even today that hasn't changed.

Even well into the 1980s, if you said you believed in God, one would assume you were religious. The delineation of "spiritual and not religious" had not made its way into the lexicon just yet. There wasn't a yoga studio on every street corner, and modern new age gurus like Deepak Chopra and Marianne Williamson were just coming onto the scene. Ram Dass pretty much held that part of the community down; he cornered the market in new thought/ancient wisdom spiritualism that encouraged young kids like me to see God in everything.

Around the same time, again thanks to the Grateful Dead, I became intimately familiar with the works of the great mythologist and author Joseph Campbell. As a young Deadhead and fledgling psychonaut, I was aware that the subcultures I was exploring had a deeper meaning to them, but I couldn't quite articulate what it was.

It wasn't just about getting high and dancing around to music; that much I knew. So when Campbell spoke about attending a Dead show in the mid '80s, it changed the entire meaning for how I was going about life. It showed me that finding deeper meaning was there to be had if you looked at it in different ways. He said:

"The Deadheads are doing the dance of life, and this, I would say, is the answer to the atom bomb . . . I had a marvelous experience two nights ago . . . The genius of these musicians, these three guitars and two wild drummers in the back . . . The central guitar, Bob Weir, just controls this crowd and when you see eight thousand kids all going up in the air together . . . Listen, this is powerful stuff! And what is it? The first thing I thought of was the Dionysian festivals, of course. This energy and these terrific instruments with electric things that zoom in . . . This is more than music. It turns something on in [the heart]. And what it turns on is life energy. This is Dionysus talking through these kids."

He continues, "It doesn't matter what the name of the God is, or whether it's a rock group or a clergy. It's somehow hitting that chord of realization of the unity of God in you all, that's a terrific thing, and it just blows the rest away."

Sidenote: One of the many amazing things about this is that Campbell was eighty-one when he went to that Dead show. It's a fine example that says we can always continue to find magic and growth at any stage of our life.

By the time I got into the Dead, they were in a late-stage career peak of both musicality and popularity. Their music and cultural impact were already legendary. Yet, there was an added sense of legitimacy due to Campbell's reflections on the Dead that was validating for the throngs of young people who followed them around the country, like myself. It was a stamp of approval that we were doing something important.

That feeling translated into my formative years of psychedelic work as well. I was around the age of eighteen when I really started to feel like I was communing with something special within the medicine.

I didn't know it then, but I sure do now. Those early experiences of psychedelic use and the introduction to lofty philosophers like Watts and Campbell made me who I am today. It firmly solidified that my life's path would be one of seeking and not of conformity. One of trial and error rather than the safe route. And most importantly, that no matter how old I am or what stage of life I find myself in, I can always continue to reinvent myself.

It certainly hasn't been a linear journey for me. I have not become enlightened, become a guru, or even have been healthy and happy all of the time. But I was given a model to look at the world through. Earlier, I mentioned my dissatisfaction with my corporate career. I almost look at this as a warning for others. It's very possible that if you go deep on a psychedelic-assisted path or one of being a mystic, you may very well wake up one day having a feeling that everything in your life doesn't feel right. It's a cautionary tale. But one that I encourage you to find out for yourself.

Reading these guys' work at the same time I was beginning my psychedelic explorations created a set of intentions that, in hindsight, turned out to be near ideal reasons for why one might want to use psychedelics in the first place: Am I staying curious? Do I desire continued growth? Do I view my life as an adventure and not a stagnant destination? And most of all, do I stay away from the societal traps that tell us that men at a certain age don't do things that aren't age appropriate?

"It's never too late to have a happy childhood," as Tom Robbins once said.

When it comes to fusing the formal understanding of Campbell's hero's journey onto the psychedelic one, it's really not that big of a leap. Let's look at some of the core principles of the hero's journey as defined by Campbell.

The hero's journey outlines a universal story structure that many myths and narratives follow, regardless of their cultural origin. Here's a simplified version of the stages of the hero's journey:

1. **The call to adventure:** The hero is called to leave their ordinary world and embark on a journey or quest. This call may come in the form of a challenge, a revelation, or an external event. Think mental health issue or personal loss, such as grief or general life dissatisfaction.

2. **Refusal of the call:** Initially, the hero may resist answering the call due to fear, doubt, or a sense of inadequacy. Maybe you come into psychedelic work being afraid or thinking that it won't work for you or that there's no hope.

3. **Meeting the mentor:** The hero encounters a mentor or guide who provides wisdom, advice, or assistance to help them on their journey. The mentor often equips the hero with the knowledge or tools they need to overcome obstacles. This may be the shaman, the psychedelic guide, or the psychedelic-assisted therapist that will help you plot the course.

4. **Crossing the threshold:** The hero makes a decisive commitment to embark on the adventure, leaving behind their familiar world and entering into the unknown. This crossing symbolizes the beginning of their transformation. Once you take the medicine, there's no going back. You can either embrace the unknown or resist the experience.

5. **Approach to the inmost cave:** The hero approaches a significant challenge or ordeal, often symbolized as an inner or outer "cave" where they must confront their deepest fears or obstacles. In the psychedelic space, you are more likely than not to confront a deep memory of your past that may frighten you, but in order to move through it, you have to look at it no matter how challenging it may be. This isn't easy work, but the end justifies the means.

6. **The ordeal:** The hero faces their greatest trial or battle, undergoing a profound transformation or revelation. This ordeal represents a crucial turning point in the hero's journey. Once you conquer that most challenging revelation in your medicine journey, you may realize that you have a renewed sense of freedom and lightness around it. That ordeal or even that most painful trauma will still be there, but with a new sense of healthy detachment.

7. **The reward (seizing the sword):** After overcoming the ordeal, the hero achieves their goal, gains new insights, or obtains a valuable reward. This reward may take various forms, such as knowledge, treasure, or enlightenment. In the psychedelic world, we call these "downloads"—the bits of information that you obtained from your journey that you can bring back with you.

8. **The road back:** The hero begins the journey back to their ordinary world, but they may face new challenges or obstacles on the return journey. This is the beginning of the integration process: How does your new life look? Are you willing to do the work? Will others understand?

9. **Resurrection:** The hero experiences a final, symbolic death and rebirth, undergoing a profound transformation or renewal. This resurrection marks the culmination of their journey and the emergence of a new, empowered self. Another stage of integration: Are you comfortable with your new self, and can you integrate it into your existing life?

10. **Return with the elixir:** The hero returns to their ordinary world, bringing back the lessons, wisdom, or gifts acquired on their journey. They may share their newfound knowledge or use it to benefit their community or society. Often, you may get so inspired as a result of

your psychedelic transformation that you may want to help others and share what you've learned. Be patient on this one. Let it take hold in you first before moving on to helping others.

Does that sound like the psychedelic experience to you? It sure does to me.

The path of self-inquiry and the commitment to an internal adventure into your own mind, heart, and soul is the essence of a successful psychedelic experience and is mystical in nature. When I discovered a neat and tidy way of juxtaposing Campbell's hero's journey archetype onto the psychedelic experience, I noticed too many similarities that I simply couldn't share.

As I've stated many times throughout this book, the efficacy of using psychedelics to treat various mental health conditions is worthy and even groundbreaking. I just fear that those who overly focus on that aspect will mistakenly leave out that the core DNA of an altered state is rooted in transcending your limited waking state of awareness and opening yourself up to a mystical reality that is filled with endless scenarios that you previously never considered. The modern psychedelic movement's discovery that these wonderfully mysterious and sacred substances can treat a variety of mental health disorders is a poignant moment in the future of mental health treatment. One that guarantees a future for these medicines through a complete re-understanding and acceptance of their place in both our present world and via their past ancient uses.

In spite of the now self-evident benefit in how these substances work on treating the less desirable parts of our humanity, the changes that occur in our brain's relationship to the issues that hold us back is not based merely on a psychological shift. The shifting spiritual relationship that psychedelics can change with ourselves and our "issues" plays just as important a role as anything else in treating our issues with these drugs.

The life lessons I learned from Campbell were to never stop learning, growing, expanding our consciousness and awareness, and conquering fears. These are the blueprints for the hero's journey of life. Of course, material world satisfaction like family, romantic love, and career are all necessary and even beautiful things to have but ultimately finding real fulfillment that keeps us interested is important.

> "What is it we are questing for? It is the fulfillment
> of that which is potential in each of us. Questing for
> it is not an ego trip; it is an adventure to bring into
> fulfillment your gift to the world, which is yourself."

—Joseph Campbell

The Awareness of Mystical States

Ancient sages, yogis, and mystics have been aware of the importance of the mystical experience for millennia. Mystical fulfillment is woven into the practice of yoga and meditation and even into some of the main Eastern religions. What I'm getting at here is that a life infused with mystical experiences was part of every culture across the globe and woven into the very fabric of the earliest psychedelic use among humans. Being mystically inclined was part of the human experience, and it was only recently that it got lost.

After the post-industrial way of life became the default system for our culture, another domino fell that was ironically counter to the nine-to-five worker mentality: free time. Automatization, convenience, and choice made it so we didn't have to spend our non-working hours procuring food and doing hard household labor. This gave way to a new generation of American mystics who pondered life, its meaning, and our relationship to the world around us. As mentioned earlier, two of the most important are Ralph Waldo Emerson and Henry David Thoreau. They are the literary and philosophical precursors to Joseph Campbell and in my estimation also helped create a window in twentieth-century culture where psychedelic explorations could take hold.

Ralph Waldo Emerson was one of the most influential figures in a new wave of American literature and philosophy. The transcendentalist movement that he was a part of emphasized individual intuition, spirituality, and the inherent goodness of people and nature. Much of his writing explored themes such as the importance of nonconformity, the value of individualism, the interconnectedness of humanity and nature, and the pursuit of truth through personal experience and intuition.

"To be yourself in a world that is constantly trying to make you something else is the greatest accomplishment" (as Emerson says) is one the finest missions that anyone can have in life and take away from a psychedelic journey.

Henry David Thoreau, who lived entirely in the nineteenth century, was perhaps one of the forebearers to the '60s counterculture that would come one hundred years after his work. In his book *Civil Disobedience*, Thoreau advocated for nonviolent resistance to unjust laws and government actions. His ideas influenced many later social and political movements, including those advocating for civil rights and environmental conservation. Many of these ideas were inspired by his connection to nature and the stillness that he found in equanimity with his own environment.

There is no evidence that Thoreau or Emerson used any kind of psychedelic plant or medicine to inspire them. I'm not even sure they knew they existed. However, as I said earlier, I do believe that the philosophical discourse they disseminated into our culture laid the groundwork for alternative forms of explorations like psychedelics and meditation, which would come later. Without these philosophies being enshrined into the American gestalt, ideas like expanding consciousness, going within, and searching for truth could have never been part of the blueprint for psychedelic research and use. They also helped usher in a form of American mysticism that isn't relegated to any one tradition or lineage and allows space for the individual to brand it for themselves. This is why it's so important, vital even, that the new wave of psychedelic popularity never loses the connection to the inherent qualities that make the experience unique.

My hope is that the growth of the psychedelic community will have a ripple effect that forces each individual who uses these compounds to take a step back, slow down, and not just look at themselves with more depth but consider their relationship to the world around them with more sensitivity and sincerity. The incessant divisions we see on TV, in our political parties, and in age-old discrimination against race, sexual orientation, and gender can be addressed at least partially by adopting routines and belief systems that include perspectives that are rooted in mysticism. That doesn't mean you need to quit your job, start wearing beads, and find a guru. All the tropes and clichés aside, we could all be better off by engaging more and more in our local communities, telling more stories to our children, buying food from local farms, and taking up hobbies rooted in art and creation.

If there's any one message I've received from sustained psychedelic use over the years is that there has to be more to life than the prescriptive formula that the American dream tells us to live up to. These drugs continuously challenge me to look deeper into the fabric of my mind.

For as long as mankind has existed, he has questioned the very nature of existence itself and sought to experience the presence of something greater. The nearly uncountable varieties of religious or spiritual experiences are very well documented, however some more so than others. Over the years, society has created a sort of ghettoization of spiritual practice that doesn't fall neatly into the big three world religions. Judeo Christianity, Islam, and Hinduism make up the vast majority of religious followers on the planet today, and due to the homogenization of those religions, their lesser known mystical offshoots have taken a backseat to a dogmatic "there is only one way" to practice approach.

Not much is known about spiritual practices aside from the three in the mainstream view of society, and when they do come up, they are branded as fringe, trendy, or culty. Even if you adhere to a formal religious practice, I encourage you to dive into the mystical cousins of those religions. Kabbalah in Judaism, Sufism in Islam, and Tantra in Hinduism are fine examples of how these ancient religions have mystical cousins. We tend to look down on rituals that aren't part of the common thread. Perhaps it's out of fear or the tendency to shun what we don't understand. A kind of spiritual xenophobia.

Witness Consciousness

There is a concept in the Eastern spiritual traditions, mainly Hindu philosophy, called "Sakshi," which simply means "witness." It is a sense of awareness that arises from spiritual practice in which you experience your mind from within. It is a sense of awareness that cannot be objectified or given meaning to, or even labeled. Again, that is another connection to successful psychedelic exploration. Ram Dass often used the term "loving awareness" as his mantra for his latter day works, and it's something that I use when guiding others in the psychedelic space.

Simply observe and view all that is transpiring with a sense of "loving awareness." Don't label it good, bad, happy, or sad. Just observe it without any attachment to the labels. That practice, much like Buddhist "witness consciousness," allows us to free ourselves from attaching negative labels to difficult events. That doesn't mean we shouldn't acknowledge the pain or suffering; it just means we can allow space for it to not weigh so heavily on our everyday life. There's a fine line between spiritual bypassing and witness consciousness. I would never want to encourage anyone to bypass their pain or compartmentalize their traumas. They all need to be acknowledged.

Every single one of us has our own story and potential for a hero's journey inside of them. If you feel a calling to explore your mind, nature, or your connection to all things, or to simply address your suffering, it should be done in a way where the clinical backdrop is not the authority of the experience. Your own voice, intuition, and deep need to be seen and heard are all that matters. Go forth with the knowing that your experience is the ultimate authority.

7

Challenging Trips

Rethinking the Narrative

"To fathom hell, or soar angelic, just take a pinch of psychedelic."

—Humphry Osmond

We've all heard stories of challenging trips. The sensationalized headline drama of a man so high on LSD that he thought he could fly so he jumped off a building. A Burning Man denizen who was so high on LSD that he walked himself into the fire, or the raver who was so high on MDMA that he went around and sexually molested women during his trip. There are countless recounts of "bad trips" attached to the potential perils of psychedelic use. While these occurrences are in the vast minority, they still have to be talked about objectively. No movement can grow if it's not honest about the risks. The pop culture references above are just a few examples. There are countless other curious souls who have gotten unintentionally destabilized due to psychedelics, mainly because their application of set and setting was poor.

As a psychedelic advocate, I have to be objective in saying that a "warning label" of sorts is essential for the proverbial bottle of LSD. What that label would say could range anywhere from "LSD-25: USE WITH EXTREME CAUTION. YOU MAY END UP THINKING FOR YOURSELF" to "LSD-25: FOR ADULT USE ONLY. AFTER USING THIS DRUG, YOU MAY WANT TO QUIT YOUR JOB."

Humor aside, even an old acid head like myself knows that drugs like LSD can produce harrowing visions and make you face your demons head-on. That is an inescapable truth behind using psychedelic drugs. Challenging experiences may be part of your journey, even with the most rigorous preparation. Hearing that may instill fear in many. However, I encourage you to open to the idea that a challenging experience may end up being one of the most valuable teaching moments and is a part of the process we must educate ourselves about.

When I was a young and impressionable teenage Deadhead, acid was a part of the social fabric, and I admit there were times I got terrified. Growing up with great psychedelic teachers and a degree of safety in that I didn't have to hide my LSD use, there were many times when the drug turned on me and flipped the world on its head, showing me parts of myself that I wasn't ready to see.

"Set and setting" are still the primary tools to apply when setting yourself up for a successful psychedelic outing (and you will learn how to create these for yourself in chapter 11). But learning to navigate these challenging experiences if and when they do happen is where the real work begins. But most importantly, never give in to the drug war propaganda that says psychedelics will make you so far gone that you'll never return. Popular narratives, media-fueled fear mongering, and misuse in the '60s due to lack of education all played a part in what we refer to as "bad trips." Some of it was real, but most of it was based in a central repository that was free from a cohesive blueprint of how drugs like LSD could and should be used. Bad trips and further destabilization certainly have occurred, but the number pales in comparison to the countless millions whose lives were forever changed for the better, thanks to the opportunity to peer through the veil that psychedelics allows.

Even Michael Pollan admitted that his later-in-life exploration into psychedelics was partly influenced by the drug war propaganda: "I waited as long as I did because I was too scared when I was young— all the post-sixties propaganda I believed—and then got too busy to devote whole days to psychedelic experience. I don't know if I ever would have tried a high-dose experience if I hadn't started interviewing people whose lives had been transformed by psychedelics."

There's no question that hearing others' stories, examining the data, and adhering to best practices can help erase the false narratives and expand our view around what exactly "bad trips" are and what to do if they should arise.

In order to examine the subject, we must direct our attention to the possible risks and the main subjective issues that can possibly lead to a challenging trip should they not be addressed beforehand. Namely, mental health afflictions, being ill prepared, impure compounds, and an unwillingness to see unsavory aspects of ourselves—what I call "looking into the cosmic mirror"—are what contribute most to the possibility of having an adverse reaction to psychedelic use.

"Bad trips," common or not, are part of the landscape of the psychedelic matrix to the extent in which you decide how much power you want to give to them. I prefer and in fact I strongly encourage anyone I work with to drop the use of the phrase "bad trip" and replace it with "challenging trip." It's much better suited to the overall purpose of this interpersonal cosmic chess match anyway. Challenging trips are just that: journeys that bring up challenging aspects of your inner workings and emotional state that may appear to freak you out when confronted with their stark existence.

The MAPS manual for working with difficult experiences says, "The most common felt threat to sanity is the feeling/experience that one is going crazy, losing one's mind, or that this will never end. This feeling/experience is supported by changing mental states and powerful (sometimes) changes in perception. Major shifts in ego/personality structure, regarding one's belief and understanding of oneself, the world, and God are common."

Part of the paradox in challenging trips is that even though they may be dark or harrowing, they still might be useful. So what is a challenging trip due to merely being shown your shadow side, and what's the result of poor planning and poor set and setting? They are two different things.

There is one realization that I've come to accept as part of the challenging trip paradigm due to working with others in the space: psychedelic drugs don't react in the same way that recreational drugs do. For instance, if you or someone you know did cocaine and did not like it, chances are they didn't like the way it made them feel. They simply didn't like the high and the person it turned them into. I find that with psychedelics, challenging experiences don't arise because someone took the drug and didn't like the way it made them feel; it's because it brought up parts of themselves, visions of an inner working, a past memory, or a frightening realization that was simply too much to look at. Adding to that, an inexperienced voyager may feel trapped inside a loop and feel that it will never end. These are very tricky realms to navigate.

Many people who work through challenging experiences describe this sensation as where the real work happens. When looking back at my own experiences, I find this to be accurate. I've been in settings so idyllic that I thought the majestic beauty of our planet would protect me from the shadow side of my inner psyche, only to find myself crying in terror at seeing the patterns and behaviors of the past that have caused me so much pain in life.

When I surrendered to the message that the spirit molecules were telling me, these types of journeys turned into an acceptance of seeing what I needed to see and not what I wanted to see. There is a profound simplicity in understanding that paradigm. It's the one that most people new to psychedelics don't fully understand, which ends up causing distress and resistance. You cannot go into a psychedelic experience thinking you can control the narrative. In fact, it's just the opposite: you must learn to surrender and listen to what's being shown. A psychedelic synesthesia if you will. And the paradox continues: the faster you surrender to the experience, good or bad, the sooner it will pass and something new will be shown to you. There is no magic formula for how to do this, but being in touch with your breath, using music as a grounding tool, and reciting mantras to yourself like "I am loved, and I am safe" can all help you navigate something challenging. Also, if you have a skilled guide alongside you, they can help steer you to safety.

In 2021, the *International Journal of Drug Policy* published a research paper entitled "Making 'Bad Trips' Good: How Users of Psychedelics Narratively Transform Challenging Trips into Valuable Experiences." The authors make the academic argument that while bad trips are certainly unpleasant, such trips are the keys to reaping the benefits of the full psychedelic spectrum.

The paper summarizes:

> Almost all participants had frightening experiences when using psychedelics, and many described these as bad trips. The key feature of a bad trip was a feeling of losing oneself or going crazy, or ego dissolution. Most users said that these experiences could be avoided by following certain rules [you'll see my suggested list later in this chapter], based on tacit knowledge in the subcultures of users. Possessing such knowledge was part of symbolic boundary work that distinguished between drug culture insiders and outsiders. Some also rejected the validity of the term bad trip altogether, arguing that such experiences reflected the lack of such competence. Finally, and most importantly, most participants argued that unpleasant experiences during bad trips had been beneficial and had sometimes given them deep existential and life-altering insights.

Within the "Making Bad Trips Good" research, it's important to note that all the participants who were surveyed had none of the preexisting conditions that may lead to a bad trip, and all of them did everything right in terms of preparation and the adherence to correct set and setting parameters. Even with those variables absent, the possibility can still occur.

And with that in mind, the *International Journal of Drug Policy* still concludes that "Bad trip experiences are common among users of psychedelics. Such experiences are often transformed into valuable experiences through storytelling. Bad trip narratives may be a potent coping mechanism for users of psychedelics in noncontrolled environments, enabling them to make sense of frightening experiences and integrate these into their life stories. Such narrative sense-making, or narrative work, facilitates the continued use of psychedelics, even after unpleasant experiences with the drugs."

Moving forward with the assumption that bad trips or challenging experiences may occur, it is still important to talk about the fundamental mistakes that can happen and why even for well-prepared, healthy people, these seemingly frightening landscapes may actually turn out to be the message one needs to hear.

Here are some examples of common types of thoughts and feelings that may occur during a challenging trip. Such experiences can appear harrowing but may be trying to show you something that's part of a larger message.

- **Trauma thoughts:** Revisiting or "reliving" the origin stories behind your trauma (i.e., war, sexual abuse, etc.).

- **Enhanced awareness:** Becoming aware of suppressed or repressed memories. These may have been buried so deep that you've forgotten them, but suddenly they are as clear as day.

- **Grief:** Feeling the pain and grief around the loss of important people in your life.

- **Thoughts about your behaviors:** Being confronted with ways you are dishonest, hypocritical, lustful, or otherwise living outside of your personal values.

- **Self-inquiry:** Becoming upset about the state of your life, the world, your partner, or what you're doing with your life.

- **Feeling out of alignment:** A sudden revelation that a major aspect of your life (work, relationships, habits, etc.) is no longer in alignment with where you want to go.

Mental Illness

It's hard to talk about mental illness in relationship to the bad trip category. That's because people who suffer from serious mental health conditions should not be using psychedelics in the first place, or at best, they should not use psychedelics until they fully understand their condition, are not currently in a mental health crisis, are free from any suicidal ideation, and are not on any psychiatric drugs. Even then, it may not be a good idea.

You might be asking yourself: but what about psychedelics and the treatment of mental health? As mentioned often previously, there is no question as to the efficacy that psychedelics have shown in treating certain forms of mental illness like depression, anxiety, and PTSD. But in the context of this chapter, it's important to understand where the line is. What constitutes the difference between severe mental illness like bipolar 1 and 2 and schizophrenia, and the everyday maladies of the human condition like those in the list above?

To make the point, there are two cases in popular culture that are worthwhile to look at, not only because they have become clichés surrounding the challenges of free-for-all psychedelic use but also because they are both well-documented accounts of how LSD assisted in triggering eventual full psyche meltdowns that were rooted in preexisting mental health conditions that were hard to identify in the 1960s. They are the tales of Syd Barrett of Pink Floyd and Brian Wilson of The Beach Boys.

I find it useful to talk about these two giants of modern music because they illustrate the classical struggle of shadow and light that exists in all of us. It just so happened that the shadow was something that neither of these two men were responsible for, and had they had better information beforehand, they could have possibly avoided the horrors that were to follow.

Syd Barrett was born in postwar England near Cambridge in 1946. Like all young men of the time, the scars of World War II Europe were impossible to miss. Ancestral trauma was a reality, and lucky for us, some of this generation channeled their pain into groundbreaking music that was chock-full of self-awareness and social commentary. John Lennon and Roger Waters come to mind. Barrett's father was not a war veteran and instead was somewhat of an intellectual, and with the aid of his mother, Syd was encouraged to take up music as a way of nurturing the bleakness of postwar England. He did so with great promise and unimaginable creativity. But there was something different about Syd. His affability and charm was frequently met with bouts of depression and an inner distance that no one had a label for at the time. When Pink Floyd got underway, his immediate talents were bright, weird, and altogether like no one else had ever seen. The quick rise to fame led Syd to capture the hearts and minds of a new England that was at the center of creating some of the greatest music the world had ever seen.

Like most of his peers, the psychedelia of the time sparked a curiosity into the magic mind drug that was LSD. When Syd introduced it into his repertoire, there was no instruction book about preexisting conditions or how to analyze one's "set" before taking the drug. The results of Syd's overuse and the subsequent lack of hard education around using it resulted in one of the great spirals of the human psyche in pop culture. The drug use, the fame, money, pressure, and underlying mental illness was too much for anyone to handle, and Syd found himself deteriorating to the point of literally being unable to function as a member of Pink Floyd. Isolated and untreated, he lingered for a few more years before vanishing into obscurity.

Later on, his bandmates admitted that Barrett was taking a drug called Mandrax, which was basically a Quaalude, to presumably soften the onset of his suspected undiagnosed schizophrenia. At the time, there was very little information on mental illnesses, and the concept of engaging in day-to-day therapy was still foreign. In 1967, having schizophrenia basically meant that you'd be relegated to a draconian psych ward. Had Syd been able to seek a more compassionate form of treatment and had someone told him that LSD might not be a good idea for his condition, things might have turned out very differently. We'll never know.

Brian Wilson, the genius of The Beach Boys, is a similar cautionary tale, but fortunately he was able to regain some of his faculties and continue to blow the world away with his talents. To this day, he identifies as having bipolar disorder and takes traditional medications to treat it. The people who are closest to Brian proclaim him to be a quiet genius but also incredibly fragile.

In the early '60s, at the height of The Beach Boys' fame, Wilson was struggling with the pressures of having to write hit songs and tour at the same time. The pressure was too much. Being the primary songwriter for The Beach Boys meant that he was responsible for the well-being of his family, who were also in the band, and staying ahead of the curve creatively. By all accounts, he exhibited a tendency to isolate and seemed to be celebrating odd behaviors, like building an indoor sandbox with a piano in it.

When he started using LSD, it seemed like he was following the recipe for creative success in the 1960s, and coupled with the rest of what was going on with him, no one really said much. After all, he wrote *Pet Sounds*! Something was working. Sadly, it didn't last. Wilson continued to spiral into almost totally unrecognizable ways that landed him in the care of a power-hungry megalomaniac doctor (Dr. Eugene Landy) who pumped his system full of drugs and kept him isolated from society. Finally, after eventually finding a compatible doctor and receiving successful treatment, he was able to resume his career as a musician. Had he been diagnosed with bipolar disorder in 1966 and properly educated on the risks of taking LSD with such a condition, he could have avoided further destabilization.

These two cases are well documented—much has been written about them. It's also fair to point out that these are extreme cases, and other factors like fame and money played a part in their eventual unraveling. Nonetheless, I hold firm that both Wilson and Barrett are very useful narratives to revisit in psychedelic lore because their downward trajectories are hallmarks in how psychedelic drugs can contribute to the further destabilization of users with severe preexisting mental health disorders. Did these drugs produce hallucinations within the minds of Wilson and Barrett? Or were there dark tapestries of horror and pain that were already there and just came to the surface?

It is understandable that there may be confusion around the words "hallucinogen" and "hallucination," both of which exist in our language in very different ways. Most medical dictionaries define a hallucinogen as "a drug that produces hallucinations," while the DSM-5 classifies "hallucinations" as one of the key diagnostic features that define psychotic disorders. Hallucinations are "perception-like experiences that occur without an external stimulus." They can be visual, auditory, olfactory, tactile, or gustatory. They exist within the context of many mental disorders like schizophrenia or dissociative identity disorder. The definition of hallucinogens can be quite confusing because hallucinogens do not cause actual hallucinations like those seen in psychotic disorders. They cause what seems to be a hallucination because they alter a person's regular sense of reality or relationship with external stimuli. Think of the walls appearing wavy, for instance. Therefore, it can be confusing when those who suffer from mental health disorders take psychedelic drugs and experience hallucinations. Which came first? What's the cause? The drug or the illness? Or both perhaps! Whatever the case may be, we can agree that the two when combined do not make a good match.

With all the information we now have in helping those who suffer from mental illness identify their condition and be provided with treatment options, we are still, very frustratingly, left with just as many questions as answers. In prior chapters, I talked about how psychedelics have revolutionized the treatment of mental health issues for possibly millions of people, and those stories are both inspiring and disruptive as they have the potential to shake up a global industry that is hell bent on pushing pills that rarely work, reaping unimaginable profits, and leaving those in need fighting for their lives.

Nonetheless, if you or a loved one are in a mental health crisis or have a severe mental illness such as bipolar disorder or schizophrenia, please understand that psychedelics may not be right for you at this time or possibly ever. Psychedelic medicines aren't for everyone, and the sooner we provide the necessary education within our society, the sooner we will see safer psychedelic use across the board.

Severe mental health issues certainly aren't the only criteria for having a challenging psychedelic experience. At any point in one's psychedelic evolution the experience can turn on you and present themes that are dark and terrifying. While no one can guarantee this won't happen, there are some actions we can take to better prepare ourselves should it happen.

Tips for Avoiding Challenging Trips

In a practical sense, it is impossible for anyone who goes into a psychedelic experience to expect not to encounter shadows, challenges, or even the darkest night of the soul. This may happen, or it may not. Here are some tips that can help you better prepare for a trip that can go in many directions.

1. First, accept the idea that challenging trips may be part of the experience and may lead to profound breakthroughs.

2. Before taking any psychedelic, look within and be completely honest with your own "set." Are you mentally

fit to be using these tools in the first place? Do you have a history of severe mental health issues? When you look in the figurative mirror, do you like what you see?

3. Educate yourself. Read everything you can about the drug you are considering using. Learn about the pros and cons.

4. Create a blueprint for your journey. Map out your healing process and what the goals are.

5. Make sure, without exception, that your "setting" is ideal and free from external harm or distractions.

6. Have a support system in place. Consider using the drug with a guide, trip sitter, or trusted friend who can support you through a potential dark corner.

7. Don't rush into it. There is no reason to rush into a psychedelic experience. Be cautious and deliberate. There's no harm in waiting until everything feels just right.

8. If a challenging experience does arise, do your very best to be deliberate around your breathing and use it to regulate your body. Also, use music and possibly even a change in scenery to reset your internal energy. None of these are guaranteed to make the challenges go away, but they can help lessen the severity.

9. DO NOT overuse any psychedelic drug. Like anything else, overuse can result in further destabilization.

I've found it can be tricky to establish a healthy "set" in terms of preparedness because one's internal climate can change from one day to the next. The unpredictability of "self" on a daily basis can affect even the most well-planned psychedelic journey. I encourage everyone to have the freedom to hit the eject button at any time, even minutes before the trip is to begin. If you feel that something is off inside of you, for whatever reason, and that it's not the right time, don't proceed. I've seen many healthy and well-intentioned people embark on rigorous planning for their journey, only to be disrupted by a personal event the day before the journey, which led to them pressing the stop button at the last minute.

Frederick Barrett from Johns Hopkins wrote in a *Personality and Individual Differences* study in 2017: "Classic hallucinogens (e.g., psilocybin and LSD) have substantial effects on perception, cognition, and emotion that can often be psychologically challenging; however, we know very little regarding the source of significant individual variability that has been observed in the frequency and intensity of challenging experiences (i.e., 'bad trips') with psychedelics . . . Conclusions: Neuroticism may contribute to the strength of challenging experiences with psychedelics in uncontrolled settings."

Barrett's quote suggests two important factors that are both nonspecific because they differ for everyone: neuroticism and uncontrolled settings.

When I was sixteen years old, I rode with a friend, who was a coworker at my teenage job at the Hard Rock Cafe in Los Angeles, up to the Cal Expo fairgrounds in Sacramento to see the annual Grateful Dead concerts. He had a classic Volkswagen bus whose purr on the open highway suggested a Kerouacian glimmer of freedom and adventure. We were on the road searching for magic wherever we could find it. The Grateful Dead were peddlers of a certain form of sonic sorcery that could wrap you around its wand and launch you into an altered state. Sure, the acid helped, but the music was even more potent.

On night two of a three-night run where fans were allowed to camp on-site at the venue, my friend, who I'll call Robert, decided to take more LSD than I did. Robert was a British bartender who was supposed to be looking after me and quickly spiraled into what at first seemed like a guy doing his best Neal Cassady impression. It then turned into something much darker and even more sinister. Keep in mind that the Grateful Dead tapestry of fans creates an almost reliable safety net, which has a tradition of supporting far-out psychedelic voyages. There are countless others on LSD, lots of colors, food in the parking lot, sympathetic brothers and sisters who all "know what it's like." Even so, things can still go wrong.

On this night, it was the very definition of an "uncontrolled setting." Immediately after the menacing "Drums/Space" portion of the set, Robert started fixating on the young pretty girls at the show. He was blazing high and started running around the entire show and then the parking lot, dry humping random legs while screaming out loud, "I WANT TO HAVE THE DEVIL'S BABY!"

At first it seemed almost comical until I realized that he wasn't going to stop. Running around endlessly screaming this demon-like mantra while physically assaulting every young woman he could find quickly turned into an emergency. And one that I could not keep up with. I too was tripping. The sheer sight of him behaving in this way made me freak out a little too but mostly froze my ability to do anything about it. Hours later, Robert came back to the campsite in tears, bloody, and afraid the cops were looking for him. What truly happened, I'll never know, but it was the first time I ever saw someone have a bad trip as a result of poor planning, too big a dose, and the risk of an uncontrolled setting. It alarmed me and showed me the potential of how quickly things can go sideways even with the best intentions.

Robert drove back to LA alone, scared and ashamed, while I made my way to other parts of the country to follow more Grateful Dead magic.

Uncontrolled settings can be volatile and unpredictable. While they aren't to blame entirely for Robert's terror trip, they did play a part in how it went from zero to one hundred instantly. Magic is a fleeting and subtle thing to capture while on psychedelics. It can happen and often does, but we must also remember the risks of letting certain elements stay unknown. The medicine has enough unpredictable messages nestled deep within its mysterious molecules that it's in our best interest to control as many external variables as possible.

Being Ill-Prepared

As a psychedelic medicine expert and spiritual guide, I recall a particular woman (who I'll call Sabrina) who had a very harrowing encounter in her very first medicine journey. Even though a licensed therapist mapped out her intentions, treatment plan, and long-term goals, it did not go as she expected, which I believe was due to not being prepared.

One red flag that was missed by everyone involved was Sabrina's sense of urgency around wanting to incorporate psychedelics into her healing. Her unbridled enthusiasm was closer to feeling rushed and impatient. And because of that, it became apparent that she did not do the required research surrounding what psychedelics can do to a person who struggles with control issues. In the end, she found the energetic purge that occurred to be helpful, but her lack of mental preparation led to an extremely challenging journey and one that she did expect would happen. This was one of those cases that, in hindsight, I wish I had encouraged her to not rush into and helped her better understand why she felt so desperate. This one journey tempered my zealotry quite a bit and showed me that the collective sense of enthusiasm and optimism around psychedelic healing isn't a bad thing, but it can often best be met with caution and patience.

Preparedness comes in many forms ranging from the establishment of a healthy "set" to an idyllic "setting" to selecting a trustworthy guide or friend. Part of the attraction to the medicalization model that we see bubbling up in the psychedelic community is that it adds a control layer to all the variables involved. A trained psychedelic-assisted therapist can control the setting and do extensive work to make sure the subject's set is in a place that is conducive to this type of work. There's no doubt that this is a plus for the medical model.

Drug Purity

Let's also talk about drug purity in reference to preparedness. Throughout this conversation, you might be wondering about adverse reactions due to impure compounds such as "street Molly" or "laced acid." I want to be clear in saying that throughout this entire book, the implication is that all the psychedelic medicines discussed are in fact pure and unadulterated. This is an assumption we as a community and I as a researcher must make.

However, I am aware that many people don't have access to pharmaceutical-grade MDMA or LSD and may rush to secure whatever they can get solely because it is the only option. This creates a myriad of problems, some of which are more complicated than others to solve on an individual level.

MDMA, in particular, experienced tremendous backlash and got labeled a Schedule 1 drug because many of the problems that occurred with it in the mid-'80s—in particular in the UK and the US—had to do with "pressed-pill Molly" that was anything but pure. The nascent rave scene created a demand so high for MDMA that the supply of pure drugs simply could not keep up. Impure pills flooded the market and by doing so changed the public perception into thinking that MDMA was not safe when in fact most people were talking about an impure and unknown dirty party drug.

There is something you can do about this. As I mentioned in chapter 2, anyone can go online and legally buy a drug testing kit that allows you to measure the purity of any substance ranging from MDMA and LSD to heroin. Harm reduction methods like these are essential steps we can take to ensure we are interacting with safe substances, and since we know we are going to do them anyway, why not make it as safe as possible? TN Scientific and DanceSafe offer affordable drug testing kits that are easy to use and accurate enough to prevent the ingestion of a foreign or harmful additive.

The rampant distribution of impure substances has wreaked havoc on all aspects of illegal drug use and the subsequent War on Drugs. Today, fentanyl causes vast amounts of overdoses for opiate users. In the psychedelic world, if you don't trust your source, the reality is you may be ingesting additives that are harmful to your physical health and may also induce the likelihood of a difficult experience.

You can never be too careful.

The Cosmic Mirror

If you ever hear anyone making false claims by saying that a psychedelic trip will always be pleasant, blissful, or revelatory, they are most likely trying to sell you a picture of bliss for their own satisfaction or sense of zealotry. I'd much rather be painted an honest picture of what may or may not happen than be sold a false narrative. Difficult confrontations, while on (usually) larger doses of psychedelics, require us to deal with parts of personalities or events from our past that we aren't ready to take an honest look at.

While it's not an enjoyable way to spend several hours, these types of experiences can also be some of the most rewarding of all the psychedelic jewels available. Most of the pain in my life has been due to substance abuse, but for reasons that most people now understand, the drug use itself was just a symptom of a much deeper pain. Psychedelic confrontations of the darkest nature helped me see the true nature of that trauma, and I'd be the first to admit that looking at my active addiction while on five grams of mushrooms is one of the least pleasant things I could possibly do with my time.

This is what I call looking in the cosmic mirror. The cosmic mirror is that place you get to where you can see your predicament exactly as it is: raw, honest, and beautiful. It's that place we get to with spiritual practice, where the universe reflects back the true nature of our humanity. Many methods and contemplative practices can also help achieve a prolonged view into this state of being. Yogis have been doing it in India for thousands of years, as have Buddhists and Christian mystics of days past.

I find myself getting very nervous when my words suggest that the use of psychedelic drugs is a method in the same way that yoga or meditation is. It isn't. Psychedelics are a powerful accelerant that, when used correctly, can speed up the process of self-inquiry and help create a malleable psycho-spiritual internal ecosystem that can make more traditional spiritual practices take an even deeper hold and become even more effective. When I get that brutally honest glimpse into the mirror that comes in the form of a psychedelic vision, I find the best way to process that vision is a prolonged meditation practice after the journey where I focus on the vision I experienced during it. This helps me process it, lean into it, and above all make friends with it. We can't run away from what makes us up—good, bad, indifferent; it's all part of what it means to be alive.

While I am weary of the plague of the constant overuse of any mind-altering substances, even psychedelics, I do see the obvious benefit that lies within the repetition of doing psychedelic work. There is no doubt that certain patterns emerge, and it can be helpful to go back in to build off of them.

Once you find yourself familiar with the chaotic floodgates of your mind during your journey, you realize that it's actually not chaotic at all; rather it's actually quite serene amid a vast state of openness where you see your thoughts for what they are: a sequential stream of ideas that reside in a queue. Gaining comfort in familiarity can only happen when you revisit the landscape a few times (probably more than that) in a set that is aimed at gaining traction with your emotional and spiritual advancement and not mired by sparkly distractions.

But there is a line. Alan Watts said, "When you get the message, hang up the phone. For psychedelic drugs are simply instruments, like microscopes, telescopes, and telephones. The biologist does not sit with eye permanently glued to the microscope, he goes away and works on what he has seen." Where the line ends between overuse and constructive repetition is up for you to decide.

When you first start swimming in the psychedelic waters, it can be so disorienting that the task of making cognitive sense out of the abstract is a tall order. When mentoring first-time psychedelic users, I always encourage them to simply try to enjoy the experience and not set their expectations to a place that resembles an "enlightenment or bust" attitude. Simply learning to sit back and observe the display of colors, thoughts, and emotions that are cascading over your consciousness takes a little time to get used to. It's not dissimilar to visiting a foreign country. Stepping out of the airport upon arriving in New Delhi, the average Westerner is overwhelmed by the sights, sounds, dirt, cows, rickshaws, smells, and colors that are everywhere. It's a complete culture shock. But once you are there for a couple of days, you begin to adapt and flow. You begin to acquiesce into the once intimidating surroundings and learn to just go with it. It's the same thing in a psychedelic journey; it takes time and experience to learn how to make the most of your time in the space. Be patient and treat it with a wide-eyed wonder and sense of curiosity.

It's prudent to simply advise the newcomer that they may or may not experience a complete 180 of their being and suggest that they simply sit back and just experience the transformative experience for what it is and nothing else. Enjoy the colors, enjoy how the sound waves morph into shapes, enjoy the physical sensations, and most importantly relinquish any attachment to how your thoughts come and go—simply observe them.

Most adults have led a full life with good and bad, pain and happiness, mistakes and triumphs. Our lives are kaleidoscopes full of polarizing tapestries of shadow and light—that is the intrinsic beauty of being human. When on psychedelics, it becomes impossible to simply focus on only the joys. It all comes into full, crystal-clear clarity in front of the cosmic mirror. While there, you face everything that makes up your life. For all its beauty and pain, you are there naked in the eyes of the One. What is so fascinating about this predicament is that you are left with two choices: bask in the complex beauty of your life or resist the sticky parts, which then result in your suffering during the trip. If you choose the latter, then you're in for a difficult ride.

When being confronted with the unflinching truth of your incarnation, you can either make peace with it in order to evolve into something better or you can choose to grasp onto the shadow with no intention of moving through it.

In one of Carl Jung's most dense explorations into unraveling one's relationship to the "self," or what he calls Aion, he says, "The shadow is a moral problem that challenges the whole ego-personality, for no one can become conscious of the shadow without considerable moral effort. To become conscious of it involves recognizing the dark aspects of the personality as present and real. This act is the essential condition for any kind of self-knowledge."

Moving through life at the warp speed that the Western world seems to require doesn't allow for much encouragement to slow down and examine all the parts of ourselves. So much emphasis, especially in the new age community, is put on the illumination of joy and our deepest innate potential. That is all fine and well-intentioned, but what tends to happen is that the relationship with balance falls out of alignment. We are taught that pure joy is available at all times, and the shadow side is merely a distraction that can be avoided if you do nothing but focus on your most authentic self.

This is most prevalent in *The Secret*'s toxic positivity prescription that became wildly popular with the release of the book by Rhonda Byrne in 2006. It says, in layman's terms, that if you focus all of your waking energy, thoughts, and actions on what it is you want to attract in life, then the results will follow almost magically. It created a ripple effect in the self-help community that extended into countless other methods ranging from yoga and meditation to breathwork and diet. There is no question that joy and abundance are worthwhile goals, but at the same time every human being who is on the path must also prepare themselves for suffering and the roots of it. The Buddha was so keen on this that he made it the first Noble Truth, which states the fundamental reality of suffering as an inherent aspect of human existence. This suffering can manifest in various forms, including physical pain, emotional distress, dissatisfaction, and the inevitable experiences of birth, aging, illness, and death.

Hindu scripture has many references to the complicated nature of all things, even God itself. When Krishna finally reveals the entirety of his divinity to Arjuna in the Bhagavad Gita, he frightens Arjuna, the tepid but curious student, who knew only of his wisdom and graceful beauty. Krishna famously says, "I am death, the destroyer of worlds!" Arjuna realized that God himself isn't any one thing, and therefore, life and duty in the material world is also not any one thing.

You cannot compartmentalize your various realities thinking that the less desirable ones will just go away.

Challenging experiences are part of the work; they're part of the deeper connection you can learn to make with yourself. Dive deep into the inner workings of everything that makes you, you. It's all part of the same stuff—just from different perspectives. I've found that the more I've been able to reflect on my shortcomings and then acknowledge them, the freer I have become. Psychedelics have played a huge part in that discovery.

"The cave you fear to enter holds the treasure you seek."

—Joseph Campbell

8

Addiction

Psychedelics and the American Epidemic

"Addictions started out like magical pets, pocket monsters. They did extraordinary tricks, showed you things you hadn't seen, were fun. But came, through some gradual dire alchemy, to make decisions for you. Eventually, they were making your most crucial life-decisions. And they were less intelligent than goldfish."

—William Gibson

If there's any one condition, affliction, or point of suffering that I have the most experience in, it's addiction. Mine was in the form of substance abuse. If this was an autobiography, I would tell my story in greater detail, but for now, it's safe to say that the hell I experienced is one that I'd want no person to ever have to go through.

The addiction crisis in America is at a level never seen before in modern history. It is affecting millions of individuals and families across the country, inducing a brand of pain, loss, and suffering that is reminiscent of any dystopian Hollywood movie. Here are some statistics that illustrate the scope and impact of the addiction crisis:

Opioid overdoses: In 2020, over 69,000 drug overdose deaths were reported in the United States, with synthetic opioids like fentanyl being a major contributor to the increase in overdose fatalities.

Alcohol use disorder: Alcohol addiction continues to be a prevalent issue. According to the National Institute on Alcohol Abuse and Alcoholism (NIAAA), approximately 20.5 million adults in the US had alcohol use disorder (AUD) in 2023.

Overall substance use disorders: The Substance Abuse and Mental Health Services Administration (SAMHSA) reported that around 20.4 million Americans aged twelve or older had a substance use disorder in 2019. This includes illicit drugs, prescription medications, and alcohol.

The impact that substance use disorders have on the American family can't be put into any common statistic. Thousands upon thousands have lost loved ones or can only visit them behind bars. And the costs associated with addiction, including health care expenses, lost productivity, criminal justice involvement, and treatment, amount to hundreds of billions of dollars annually.

My addiction story included jails, institutions, and homelessness. No matter how hard I tried to do it differently, I always ended up there. Those are realities of active addiction that you never think would happen to you, and once you get there, it's hard to imagine pulling yourself out. They are the bleakest and most hopeless stops of our civilization. When you arrive, it's as if you've been welcomed into some form of purgatory on earth. You realize that you aren't dead, but being a resident in any of these places is barely being alive.

What's worse than finding yourself homeless or in county jail is that moment after the drugs have left your system and you wake up realizing all the damage you've caused. The damage I did to myself felt terrible, yes, but the damage I caused to others was far more potent. For the first couple of weeks, I could barely look in the mirror knowing there was a part of me, when activated by addiction, that would stoop to such desperate lows of depravity, dishonesty, and mayhem. I didn't like knowing that person was in there and could unleash himself if not taken care of. Healing took a long, long time. And I can't say with certainty that it will ever be complete—it's a lifelong process.

When you first get into recovery and put together some clean time, most people (certainly not all) welcome you back with warm arms and say, "I'm so glad that you're okay!" But when you relapse, it turns very quickly into "Get away from me!" Addiction is hard to understand for people who have had no personal experience with it. From what others have told me, it feels opaque because most forms of addiction are self-inflicted. One makes the choice to use heroin or smoke crack or become bulimic. The reality of it is, of course, far more nuanced than that. It would be so simple if it were just one bad choice that spiraled out of control.

Years of unprocessed trauma build up endless amounts of somatic and emotional pain that have no outlet. When you become so unregulated and unable to live life on life's terms and then discover that a temporary numbing agent exists, it doesn't seem too crazy at that moment to try it. I know that sounds insane to some, but it's the mindset for most when they make the choice to pick up that first hit.

With substance abuse, there is also a physiological response to the drug when putting it into one's body, often referred to as the lack of an "off switch." I learned the hard way that I have no off switch when opiates are put into my body. My brain's inability to regulate dopamine levels, combined with all the unprocessed trauma, created a perfect storm that turned into a Category 5 hurricane of "I need more."

Dr. Gabor Maté, a renowned addiction expert and trauma specialist, has provided powerful insights into the nature of addiction. He said, "Not all addictions are rooted in abuse or trauma, but I do believe they can all be traced to painful experiences." I really don't know for certain, nor does anyone else, which part factors more into addiction: the physiological predisposition or the high amounts of unprocessed trauma. I can't say for certain that if I had done a significant amount of trauma healing before I picked up the first drug that I would have not continued to use.

Maté's perspective is that addiction often stems from deeper emotional pain, trauma, or unresolved issues rather than simply being a result of the substance or behavior itself. He emphasizes the importance of understanding the underlying causes and psychological factors that drive addictive behaviors, advocating for a compassionate and holistic approach to addressing addiction.

The twelve-step-based recovery that originated with Alcoholics Anonymous (AA) definitely put into play a method for self-inquiry, but it also put a lot of emphasis on the community aspect of healing. Group meetings and finding others who suffer from the same affliction somehow create an atmosphere of being in it together. I found a lot of healing and resonance in Narcotics Anonymous (NA). I found a group of wonderful people and a sponsor who helped me change my life. I can't thank them enough for their unconditional love and support during my ups and downs; they were always there for me.

When I first got into recovery, the cause of my deeper emotional pain was a mystery to me. I started to scratch the surface through my active participation in the twelve steps, meditation, and lots of psychotherapy, but I still wasn't able to get a clear enough picture that kept me from relapsing. After years of clean time and involvement in the recovery community, I ended up relapsing. Part of it was due to a surgery I had that led to me abusing my pain medications, but again, I came to learn that the main part of it was a deeper mirror that I had yet to look in.

I got clean again when I started to reinvestigate my passion for Eastern mysticism and practice, namely yoga and meditation. That really started to stir things up. It culminated in my visit to Ram Dass in Maui, and from that moment on, my life changed. The details and inspiration of all that is, again, best suited for my autobiography. But the landscape was wide open. My mind was more open than it had ever been. I was so hungry for more information, answers, and for a path that could help it all make sense. I started coming to the psychedelic community around the same time and paid special attention to many stories that I heard about people who found an even deeper connection to their addiction recovery through the use of psychedelics. Some were personal stories from friends, and others were based in research and clinical trials. You have to understand that at that time I was still indoctrinated to the idea that recovery meant complete abstinence and that you could not treat the dependence of one drug with another drug. What I failed to see was that my drug dependence was just a symptom and that I wasn't treating that. I was treating my trauma—the real deep, dark, scary traumas that I was never fully ready to look at.

One afternoon in Maui, on the red sand beach, I decided to give psilocybin mushrooms a try after a nine-year break from them. I was once again newly sober and thought I had nothing to lose. I was well-versed in the principles of set, setting, and dosage and had over two hundred trips under my belt. I went forth on an experience that would change my life forever and have me look at my addiction in an entirely new way.

The mushroom projected what I could only describe as the "movie of me." Except it was two movies of me playing simultaneously on screens next to one another. One was the me that was in active addiction—afraid, desperate, and dishonest. That person would go to any lengths to get high. I mean that literally. The other movie was the projection of myself that was free from the bondages of addiction and suffering—completely in my dharma, living a life of purpose and joy. The darker movie's energy seeped into my mind as I was lying on the beach and created an energetic frequency so repulsive that all I wanted was to get as far away from that as possible. The more gentle movie was a version of Self not yet created but I knew was possible. The two different energies were pinging off each other, fighting for space. I felt that spirit was telling me I had a choice.

Later on during the trip, I made the choice to invite in the more loving version of me while merely observing the shadow side. Once I chose to bear witness to the part of myself that became addicted to drugs, I was able to be shown some of the reasons why it happened in the first place. I always thought trauma was something for other people. It was something that war vets or sexual abuse survivors had. It wasn't something an upper-middle-class kid from a famous household had the right to have.

There's a profound lesson in that small but powerful bit of learning.

Trauma is not a competition. It's not relegated to only the most severe and obvious forms. If you're able to look deep enough, you might find that you too have an event or some childhood neglect that you've forgotten about, or maybe you made a decision that led to dire consequences. These are just a few of the events that can happen in life that could have rooted themselves so deeply into your body and psyche that some traumatic residue remains.

I was able to see clearly the pain of my parents' divorce and the wild oddity of growing up the way I did, and while it did give me so much, it also lacked any real foundational instructions for life. I was able to feel the pain of my father's death and how it left me alone, afraid, and, most importantly, with no idea of who I was as a person. I was his son, not an independent person with his own thoughts and ideas. This was a terrible shock for me to come to terms with. I'm not sure I've ever had a single psychedelic journey that taught me so much. It was a profound experience full of pain and terror but ultimately led to a sense of freedom and honesty in levels never before imagined. My addiction no longer needed to define me. Yes, somewhere inside of me it remains, but the subtle beauty of embracing my own dharmic truth is an option that I hope I've done my best to live up to ever since.

There was a strange, unsettling, but very warm comfort when I revisited the mushroom that time and found it to heal something so painful. I had so much experience in the psychedelic space, but because most of it was in my young adulthood and youth, I never had any reason to turn the mirror so far onto myself.

Psychedelics and Addiction

Using psychedelics as a treatment for addiction is nothing new. In fact, one of the earliest well-studied potential uses for LSD and one of the earliest examples of psychedelic-assisted therapy was its use as a treatment for alcoholism in the 1950s. The model for how a client interacts with the therapist in a clinical setting is still used today, albeit things aren't as stiff as they were in the '50s. This period marked a time of exploration into the therapeutic potential of psychedelics, including LSD, for various mental health conditions—addiction being one of them.

Research conducted during this era, notably by psychiatrist Dr. Humphry Osmond and others, explored the effects of LSD on individuals struggling with alcohol addiction. The rationale behind using LSD for alcoholism treatment was based on the belief that the drug's psychedelic experience might lead to profound insights, spiritual experiences, and psychological breakthroughs that could help individuals address underlying issues contributing to their addiction.

One of the key proponents of LSD-assisted therapy for alcoholism was Dr. Osmond, who, along with Dr. Abram Hoffer, conducted studies involving LSD sessions for alcoholics. They reported anecdotal evidence of some participants experiencing reduced cravings, increased self-awareness, and insights into the root causes of their addiction following LSD sessions. Some individuals reported having profound experiences that led to shifts in their perspectives, attitudes, and behaviors related to alcohol use. The therapeutic approach typically involved administering LSD in a controlled and supportive environment, accompanied by psychotherapy sessions before, during, and after the LSD experience. These sessions aimed to facilitate introspection, emotional processing, and self-reflection to help individuals confront and resolve psychological issues underlying their addiction.

Most famously Bill Wilson, the cofounder of Alcoholics Anonymous, also used LSD to take a deeper look into the nature of alcoholism and ego. Wilson shared his thoughts on how LSD might serve spirituality in a 1958 letter to Sam Shoemaker. "[LSD] seems to have the result of sharply reducing the forces of the ego," Bill noted, pointing out the "generally acknowledged fact in spiritual development that ego reduction makes the influx of God's grace possible . . . [LSD] will never take the place of any of the existing means by which we can reduce the ego, and keep it reduced."

In a letter Wilson wrote to Carl Jung, the legendary Swiss psychologist, he said, "Some of my AA friends and I have taken the material [LSD] frequently and with much benefit," adding that the powerful psychedelic drug sparks "a great broadening and deepening and heightening of consciousness."

It became apparent, however, that the rise in popularity of LSD with the counterculture of the '60s put a damper on Wilson's use of the drug. It also created a deep schism within the AA community on the definition of what it means to be "sober." For reasons that I personally understand, the AA community tended to lean on the idea that complete abstinence from all mind- and mood-altering chemicals was necessary to achieve and maintain long-term sobriety. The model for complete abstinence within the twelve-step community became the standard for all the substance abuse fellowships to follow. AA, NA, Cocaine Anonymous (CA), and Crystal Meth Anonymous (CMA) all became very active communities around the world that would never allow, in the slightest, for the disease of addiction to be looked at through another lens that may include psychedelic therapy. In the late '90s, when I first got introduced to NA, even the vague mention that someone could find deeper relief with the aid of psychedelic-assisted therapy was a nonstarter. No one wanted to hear it, and even today, while the views are expanding, it's still a hot button issue.

The funny thing is that these things have a way of sorting themselves out. The rise in popularity of psychedelic research combined with the rise of the addiction epidemic in America created two different paths that I feel were destined to meet. The sheer number of people who have had positive psychedelic experiences but also suffered from addiction issues landed themselves in twelve-step fellowships where they noticed a lack of acceptance and understanding.

The great and dearly departed Ralph Metzner wrote a blazingly insightful (but sometimes dense) essay called "Addiction and Transcendence as Altered States of Consciousness." In the opening lines he wrote, "To an unbiased observer of human nature, it would appear that addictions, compulsions, and attachments are a normal and inevitable part of human experience. To this same observer, a visitor from another world perhaps, it would probably also be evident that searching for transcendence, for expanded or heightened states of consciousness, is an equally pervasive and natural human activity."

Psychedelics and Recovery

Because of mankind's quest for seeking transcendent states of consciousness in combination with its tendency to get addicted, we've seen a great change in the cultural landscape around addiction and psychedelics. The numbers of both camps became so large that there are now twelve-step organizations and non-twelve-step recovery groups that have made the inclusiveness of psychedelics part of their doctrine.

One such group is Psychedelic Recovery based in San Francisco and founded by a very passionate and somewhat evangelistic woman named Danielle Nova. Psychedelic Recovery's mission statement states, "Our mission is to shift the paradigm around how we understand, heal, and treat addiction to a framework based in self-love, empowerment, and transformation. We are a group of peers in recovery that believe that psychedelics and plant medicines can help us dissolve addictive patterns that we are ready to release from our lives.

We gather regularly to support one another to effectively understand and integrate these life-changing tools."

Part of Nova's foundation for this group was based in part on the scorn and judgment she felt from AA; therefore, Psychedelic Recovery does not use the twelve steps as part of their healing modality. I asked Danielle about what I see as the main issue with psychedelic-aided recovery groups: presenting the notion that we can treat dependence of one drug with the aid of another and how she sees that problem unfolding.

She said, "I believe that psychedelics, if used with intention, respect, reverence, and caution, can play an active role in helping people treat drug dependency and help individuals sustain long-term recovery. It is important to know that much of the work of these medicines is through the integration process, embodying the realizations that come from the psychedelic experience, and creating actionable steps to change and transform our lives."

Danielle's statement paints a clear picture of what highly intentional psychedelic use could look like and the difference between recreational and intentional use. If we follow a protocol and treat the drug with reverence, we can turn the realizations into action steps that are practical. I'd also add that when you use psychedelics for very serious reasons, such as taking a look at your addiction, the journey is almost bound to be challenging and insightful. It won't be full of fairies and rainbows. The older I get and the more I take serious issues into my psychedelic use, the more intense and difficult the trip is.

As my father Timothy once said, "Psychedelics are confrontational drugs, not escapist ones." That couldn't be more accurate when they are used for very specific reasons and not just casually dosing at a Dead show.

In addition to Psychedelic Recovery, there is also a twelve-step based, noncentral meeting collective called Psychedelics in Recovery. Yes, a one-word difference in the names in case you are Googling it. They use the twelve steps in accordance with the traditional way (sponsor/sponsee relationship) but allow for a more permissive view of abstinence by including the use of psychedelics as sacred sacraments for healing.

I'm not sure that the greater AA and NA communities will ever get to a point where they see the use of, say, Ayahuasca in a ceremonial setting as anything but a relapse. I understand why they say refraining from all drugs is essential based on the idea that using one drug will later lead to the use of your drug of choice, but ultimately I find the entire stance on it to be utterly hypocritical and an example of establishment propaganda.

There are countless members of these fellowships who are on psychiatric medications and benzodiazepines prescribed by a doctor. Whether or not these prescriptions are valid and needed for mental health issues isn't the point. The idea that a drug is only okay to take if it's prescribed and therefore accepted by the mainstream medical establishment is something that the twelve-step community should take a cold, hard look at. It is insulting as it is narrow-minded and archaic. Taking a sacrament with the aid of a shaman or a trained facilitator in a controlled setting with a very specific realm of intentions is a brave and useful thing to consider doing. In the context of recovery, I would even take it a step further and say that it's an embodiment of the third and eleventh steps, which are all about developing a relationship with a God of "your understanding."

If you are stable, intentional, and cautious, I can't think of a more noble and righteous way to get closer to an idea of a God that both serves you and enables you to develop a real and long-lasting personal relationship with. I have no qualms in whichever method anyone chooses that gets them in touch with this age-old quest of the human spirit.

So, how can we say that a doctor giving you benzos is okay, but a healer giving you Ayahuasca is not? Not only is that a great contradiction, but it is also symptomatic of the War on Drugs propaganda-filled narratives that have permeated modern culture. There is no War on Drugs. There is a war on some drugs that are taken by people we don't like. And these dangerous ideas should have no place in what road someone chooses to heal themselves.

Recommendations and Cautionary Disclaimer

While I do maintain that psychedelic drugs have helped me and countless others in healing their addiction, any addict who is considering this path should tread with great caution. I am not a medical professional nor a trained addiction expert. I can only share my personal experience from my own body and in helping others. I therefore recommend the following criteria if you are a recovering addict who is thinking about incorporating psychedelics into their wellness regimen.

- Get clean and sober first. Try to develop a fair amount of sobriety before rushing to the aid of psychedelics. How long that may be is up to you. Being stable and back on your feet can only help the psychedelic better serve you.

- Treat your psychedelic work as a sacramental and ceremonial offering. Do not do this work as cause for mindless recreational use.

- Using psychedelics to aid in your addiction healing is best done with a trained facilitator, shaman, or therapist. Do not go at it alone.

- Go within and be honest about your intentions: Are you looking to truly heal and go deeper into the root cause of your addiction? Or are you just looking to get high? Only you can answer that.

Psychedelics and Withdrawal

In addition to ongoing and sustained healing within the addiction process, there has also been a tremendous amount of research done on how psychedelics can aid in the withdrawal process. Certain psychedelics can snap people out of the painful and extended detox process and help with long-term withdrawal symptoms. Most notably, ibogaine can snap a person out of heroin addiction and remove most of the process of withdrawal.

Ibogaine is a psychoactive alkaloid derived from the root bark of the iboga plant, native to certain regions in West Africa. It has gained a lot of traction for its potential in treating addiction, including heroin withdrawal, due to its complex pharmacological effects on the brain and the nervous system. Iboga and ibogaine are two slightly different things. Iboga is primarily used in ceremonial rituals by the Bwiti tribes of Western Africa, mainly in Gabon. Their medicine ceremonies are rich with polyrhythmic explorations into controlled chaos with a touch of beauty. Most Westerners who get invited in come back feeling like they time traveled through some sacred portal of millennia past.

Ibogaine has its essence in the natural iboga plant but goes through a laboratory-aided transformation. As a result, ibogaine is often produced via semi-synthesis starting from voacangine. Conversion of voacangine to ibogaine generally requires a two-step protocol involving saponification of the C16 methyl ester followed by acidification and heating to induce decarboxylation. The complicated chemical and neuropharmacology behind it gives us some indications on why it may help individuals going through heroin withdrawal.

Ibogaine interacts with various neurotransmitter systems in the brain, including serotonin, dopamine, and opioid receptors. It's believed to modulate these systems, potentially alleviating withdrawal symptoms and reducing cravings associated with opioid dependence. Chronic opioid use alters the brain's neurochemistry and neural pathways. Ibogaine is thought to induce neuroplasticity and neurogenesis, potentially resetting or reorganizing these pathways. This effect might contribute to reducing withdrawal symptoms and cravings by altering the brain's response to opioids. The notable part about this chemical phenomenon is that it can knock out opiate dependence in hours as opposed to weeks.

But the catch is you also have to go through a wildly intense and often hellish trip to get there. So yes, you can get off opiates, but you are also signing up for one of the most relentless psycho-spiritual exorcism types of psychedelic journeys around. This profound altered state of consciousness may lead to introspection, insights, and emotional processing, allowing individuals to confront underlying psychological issues contributing to addiction.

Danielle Nova shared her thoughts on why this is valuable for the addict seeking recovery: "Psychedelics can create neurogenesis in the brain and create new pathways to teach people how to live without a dependency to a substance or behavior. They can help people create new healthy rituals and practices in a person's life. They helped me develop an intimate relationship with myself and find empowerment within. Through accessing the subconscious mind through the use of psychedelics, we can learn how to remove triggers and heal the root of the trauma, which led us to self-soothe in the first place."

Ibogaine, while illegal in the US, is legally available in clinics in Mexico, many of which profess to have success rates that are far beyond traditional detox facilities. Felipe Malacara, MD, the chief clinical operations director at Beond (an ibogaine clinic in Cancun, Mexico), said, "I have treated more than two thousand patients with ibogaine over seventeen years, and the relapse rate is about 50 percent in the long term, but around 85 percent of people leave the clinic without withdrawals and cravings."

If you look at Dr. Malacara's statistical breakdown, you will notice the amazingly high success rate on the actual detox process but a very modest success rate on long-term recovery. That's important to isolate because any addict in recovery (like myself) will tell you that there is no one short-term method, event, or procedure that will keep you clean and sober. Long-lasting recovery is best achieved by looking at your life moving forward as a holistic wellness routine. Meetings, spiritual practice, therapy, yoga, meditation, and yes, psychedelics can all play a part in a personalized combination of structure and routine that works for each individual person.

Ibogaine, if implemented in the US, would require some rigorous regulation and safety protocol standards before being rolled out.

Even with detox success rates so high, the trip itself isn't for everyone. However, under proper supervision and with the right screening, it could only bolster the nation's toolset in treating substance abuse.

No one person's recovery will look the same as anyone else's. This is why I again stress the importance of expanding our cultural and practical world view on what methods may be helpful for some, like psychedelics. The reality of it is that no one method works 100 percent of the time, so why not provide as many options as possible to allow for this crisis to get some relief?

9

Walking Each Other Home

Death, Dying, and Grief

"Death is perfectly safe. It's like taking off a tight shoe."

—Ram Dass

There's an immediate parallel between the psychedelic experience and dying. When I witness someone having a high-dose psychedelic experience—meaning those so big that they challenge the very nature of your waking reality and dissolve the ego into pure consciousness—two phrases are most commonly spoken: "I've seen the face of God!" and "Holy shit. I'm dying!"

Time and time again, I've heard people (and myself) shout out to the heavens that they are dying when the mushroom teacher takes over the mind's control mechanisms and forces the voyager to just lie back and receive what's being shown. Those are the moments when the identity of our avatar fades away and all we are left with is an ephemeral plane of energy streaming through our minds and hearts. I suspect that is very similar to what it feels like to die.

Dr. Rick Strassman, in his book *DMT: The Spirit Molecule*, suggests that our brains' natural repository of DMT gets released when we die. While there is no hard science to support that idea, anyone who has experienced "death" while on a large-dose psychedelic journey would support the claim. It's no wonder that the study of using psychedelics to ease the anxiety around death and dying are bearing such fruitful results. The psychedelic experience is tailor-made to examine the thin veil between life and death.

Leary, Alpert, and Metzner's 1964 book *The Psychedelic Experience* took on this connection quite literally. It juxtaposed the onset of the psychedelic trip against *The Tibetan Book of the Dead*, which is an ancient text that views the ascension into death as traversing six different bardos that ultimately land you in moksha, or liberation. It was a very intuitive and ultimately spiritual lens to look at the psychedelic journey through.

What I always find so challenging in my own worldview is that no matter how spiritual I think I am, death is something I can never quite make peace with and it leaves a gaping hole in my heart whenever it happens. With Ram Dass being my primary teacher, you'd think I would have made a little more progress.

On some days I have. I can feel the serene and peaceful beauty of knowing that we are all "walking each other home" and that everyone I've lost is right beside me keeping me company as I progress on the path of life. But on other days, I miss the people and animal friends (yes, my pets) that I've lost something fierce. It can permeate my every waking thought, conjuring up memories of the joy and love we experienced on the plane of the material world. Our best moments in life are usually ones that have been experienced with others. That's part of the magic of being alive—that bond that is formed when you connect with another in a way that is similar to the way that you view the world. Realizing that we are not alone provides me with so much comfort. In writing these pages, I find myself tearing up at recalling some of those people and furry friends.

The fear of being alone terrifies me as I suspect it does most of us. Loneliness is a painful void that I see when I look in people's eyes. I can see the quiet desperation seeping out of someone's heart when all they want is to be seen and understood. It's a terrible thing when you lose that person who fills that void. But the reality of it is that "no one here gets out alive," to echo Jim Morrison. I always loved Ram Dass's sense of conviction when he spoke about the death and dying process. I believed that he believed what he was saying with every ounce of his soul and that if I could just get a sliver of that belief, then I too would find peace when remembering the loss of a loved one.

The night I watched my father transition from this world to the next, I became convinced that something does happen to us when we die, that we don't just turn to nothing. And at the same time, the incredible sadness that goes with the transition is a sadness that has no equal. Witnessing the moment of his last breath was something that felt transcendental, impermanent, and not based in finality. What little energy was left in his body moved somewhere else; it turned into an energetic presence that swirled around the room in bright colors until the peak frenzy just vanished into thin air.

What happens after we die is such a mysterious and potent part of the human experience and has become the foundation for every major world religion. Heaven, hell, purgatory, or reincarnation. Take your pick. I don't think any of us truly know.

When Timothy found out he was dying, the first call he made was to Ram Dass. After all of these years, I now realize two things perplexing about that decision. One, it was an odd thing to do for a self-proclaimed philosophical materialist, and two, it indicated that Timothy was far more spiritual than he let on. The latter was a total threat to his reputation, but lo and behold, funny things can happen when we are desperate. He made that call because he knew Ram Dass approached death and dying with a perspective that transcends fear, acknowledging the impermanence of life while emphasizing the continuity of consciousness beyond physical existence. And Timothy certainly wanted to grasp onto the notion that there must be something more after we die.

Ram Dass centered on the notion of recognizing the eternal nature of the soul and the interconnectedness of all beings, providing comfort and insight into the transition from life to death. And for months after that first call, Timothy was dancing and singing glorious praises to what he called "sneak peaks," or those little glimpses into the unknown that he fell into prior to leaving his body. Indeed, he was showing us that it was "perfectly safe."

He was surrounded by loved ones at the moment of his final breath and did a hero's job at preparing us for the inevitable. I'm very fortunate that at the age of only twenty-two, I was given a model for how to die with such grace and dignity. And in case you're wondering, Timothy was not on LSD when he died. However, Aldous Huxley was!

In her memoir *This Timeless Moment*, Laura Huxley, Aldous's wife (and visionary in her own right) described how her husband took LSD as he died. "He had taken this moksha medicine in which he believed. Once again he was doing what he had written in *Island*, and I had the feeling that he was interested and relieved and quiet."

> After half an hour, the expression on his face began to change a little, and I asked him if he felt the effect of LSD, and he indicated no. Yet, I think that something had taken place already. This was one of Aldous's characteristics. He would always delay acknowledging the effect of any medicine, even when the effect was quite certainly there, unless the effect was very, very strong, he would say no. Now, the expression on his face was beginning to look as it did every time that he had the moksha medicine, when this immense expression of complete bliss and love would come over him . . . Then I began to talk to him, saying, "Light and free." Some of these things

I told him at night in these last few weeks before he would go to sleep, and now I said it more convincingly, more intensely—"Go, go, let go, darling; forward and up. You are going forward and up; you are going towards the light. Willingly and consciously you are going, willingly and consciously, and you are doing this beautifully; you are doing this so beautifully. You are going towards the light; you are going towards a greater love; you are going forward and up. It is so easy; it is so beautiful. You are doing it so beautifully, so easily. Light and free. Forward and up . . . Easy, easy, and you are doing this willingly and consciously and beautifully. Going forward and up, light and free, forward and up towards the light, into the light, into complete love." . . . The twitching stopped, the breathing became slower and slower, and there was absolutely not the slightest indication of contraction or struggle. It was just that the breathing became slower—and slower—and slower, and at five-twenty the breathing stopped. [Text sourced from organism.earth/library/document/a-beautiful-death.]

Easing End-of-Life Anxiety: Landmark Research

Decades later, we are seeing some of that work continue in more formal and rigorous studies that are focused on using psychedelic drugs to ease end-of-life anxiety. One example is Dr. Anthony Bossis, who is the co-lead at the NYU department of psychedelic research. I find Dr. Bossis to be a mystic who is hiding out as a psychologist at an academic institution. He's an avid meditator and Deadhead who also happens to be a clinical psychologist. Pretty much the perfect person to lead these sorts of studies.

The work he's led on using psilocybin to address end-of-life anxiety has contributed significantly to the growing body of research on not just end-of-life anxiety but psychedelic-assisted therapy as a whole.

If you watch his TED Talk, you'll find it to be more of a commentary on how the medical establishment should provide cancer patients access to a mystical experience than it is an exploration into hard data. He emphasizes the qualities of mystical psilocybin experiences that include the unity effect, noetic consciousness, and the necessity of encouraging his patients to use their time on psilocybin to "go within."

The studies have combined the potential of psilocybin-assisted therapy with the mystery around death, which has resulted in alleviating anxiety, depression, and existential distress in individuals facing life-threatening illnesses, particularly those nearing the end of their lives. The trials, like most of the other modern ones out there, involved a carefully controlled setting where participants received psilocybin in conjunction with psychological support and therapy sessions. These brave cancer patients reported profound and transformative experiences during the sessions characterized by a sense of unity, transcendence, and altered perception of time. Many described these experiences as spiritually significant, providing a deeper understanding of life, death, and their personal existence.

The NYU studies observed a significant reduction in anxiety and depression among participants following psilocybin-assisted therapy sessions. Dr. Bossis said, "A single dose of psilocybin produced sustained and immediate reduction in anxiety and depression . . . and 80 percent of the participants reported the same reduction six months later." Additionally, participants often reported an improved quality of life, enhanced emotional well-being, and an increased sense of acceptance and peace regarding their mortality after undergoing psilocybin-assisted therapy.

The findings from these NYU studies have influenced ongoing research efforts exploring the use of psychedelics in palliative care and end-of-life settings, contributing to a broader understanding of how these substances might offer therapeutic benefits to individuals facing existential anxiety and distress associated with terminal illnesses. Using psychedelics to ease end-of-life anxiety has also left the research lab and helped expand a rather large network of "underground" psychedelic death doulas who are a cross between witchy priestesses trained in the art of easing death transition and shaman-like medicine workers who are skilled psychedelic facilitators. It's a fascinating multidisciplinary practice that addresses the core need for us to rethink dignity around the dying process. There is even a psychedelic end-of-life doula certification program run out of Jamaica (where mushrooms are legal) by a group called the Diaspora Psychedelic Society.

Death, dying, and the industry that supports it has changed a lot over the years. Hospice care and compassionate views on quality of life are becoming more and more common than the modern medicine establishment's tendency to keep people "alive" on machines hoping for a miracle. And death doulas are becoming less and less fringe, and they're even being brought into hospices all around the country. That's a good thing. The stigma around death being a cold and sterile business that takes place in hospitals rather than hospices or at home is changing, and the ripple effects are numerous. I'm hopeful that the more people who get turned on to the idea that death is a sacred act of dignity, the more we will collectively view life as something sacred and not a capitalistic-fueled rush to see who has amassed more stuff in the end. My father taught me at a young age that the dying process should be done on terms that ensure quality of life and that celebrate the time we had on this planet. For a young man, it was a lesson well received.

Perhaps it's because of the mysterious nature of transitioning to the next plane and the dependency we put on having our loved ones next to us throughout this journey we call life that the anxiety and fear around all parts of death and the dying process runs so rampant in our culture.

Psychedelics, Grief, and Loss

Finally, in summarizing the ever-expanding world of where death and dying meet the psychedelic experience, I want to share a compelling story.

Jane, a woman who came to me for psychedelic guidance, was stricken with grief so paralyzing that her otherwise full life was put on hold. Jane had a very successful career, many hobbies, and was in excellent health for a fifty-five-year-old woman. About nine months prior to coming to see me, her husband of twenty-three years, Robert, had passed away due to a sudden heart attack. He literally left the material world in an instant while in the middle of a doubles tennis match they were playing with two of their closest friends. He died suddenly and without any warning.

After months of what she described as living a "zombie life," she ran out of answers for how to process her grief. She watched Ram Dass's videos, read books, and even spoke to a psychic. Nothing really filled that hole in her heart or brought her closer to the idea that her husband's memory could in fact live on. She stumbled upon Michael Pollan's *How to Change Your Mind* not so much because she was interested in psychedelics but because it was a bestseller and just seemed like an interesting thing to read while she was figuring what to do with her life. The book's impact was so great that she got lost in a YouTube rabbit hole and stumbled upon the aforementioned Dr. Anthony Bossis's TED Talk. That lecture and the research it presents is aimed at giving psilocybin to people who are dying and not to the bereaved themselves, but her intuition told her that was just a minor detail. She became immediately curious if the psychedelic experience could alter her perception of Robert's transition and help her find a way to make it make sense.

After much searching, she found me and made the trip from Chicago to California to do a medicine session with only one intention in mind: heal her grief. Jane was fastidious in her prep work, dotting every I and crossing every T. Her pre-journey written work was long, vulnerable, and left no details out. She took the work incredibly seriously. Because she was brand-new to psychedelics, I advised her to start slow and build up to a higher dose that would reveal more and more over time. She was adamant that was not the path she wanted to go on. She had time for one journey and wanted to make the most of it. So, after much back and forth, we agreed on a dose of four grams of Penis Envy mushrooms, which are very strong.

As the journey began and the medicine started to take hold, it was as if I was observing an experienced psychonaut on their twentieth journey. There was no resistance, no shaking, no fear—just pure surrender to the beauty that was unfolding. I gave her a couple of voice prompts about ninety minutes into the session and was met with silence. She was beyond words. After the third or fourth attempt, I gently encouraged her to send some love to Robert and invite him into the space. That clicked. For the next two hours, there were cycles of mantra-like phrases of "Robert, I love you so much. I hope you're happier now" over and over again.

Then, there was "Robert! I'm right here! I miss you so much. Why did you leave me?"

"Oh, that makes sense. I thought you left me. You didn't. I see that now. You're right here."

"But honey, the house is so empty. What should I do?"

"Okay, I'll do that, and I'm okay. I know that you'll be right here, every step of the way."

Robert's answers were something I couldn't hear, but what I've shared here are direct quotes from Jane's session. Somehow the mushroom session freed her from the trap of making his loss all about her missing him and instead turned into him being free. The plant teacher spoke to her in actual words and created a space for her to forge a new way of dealing with Robert's passing.

Not only was her relationship with the specific situation now different, her overall relationship with death and dying was forever changed. It was as if I witnessed someone on the fast track to spiritual growth. I witnessed someone who was admittedly not a very spiritual person prior to the mushroom ceremony almost turn into a buddha of sorts! She was wise, calm, and in acceptance. Jane's experience under my guidance certainly doesn't warrant a conclusive medical study, but it does show how an average person with everyday problems can have a successful, life-changing experience on psilocybin as a result of rigorous pre-session planning and very clear intention setting.

More than two years later (at the time of me writing this), she still checks in and expresses that she misses the physical presence of her husband of twenty-three years but that she knows leaving the body is not permanent. She feels Robert's presence every day and is free from the bondage of grief.

10

Set, Setting, and Sustainability

A New Model for Efficacy and Transformation

"Know thyself."

—Socrates

Nearly anyone who has used psychedelic drugs (or anyone about to) is probably familiar with the now ubiquitous concept of "set and setting." The term, I'm proud to say, came from my father's work when he was at Harvard in the early '60s. Of all his work on the power and potential of psychedelics, this framework for mapping out a safe and effective journey has stood the test of time and is still being used sixty years later.

The phrase "set and setting" came into the psychedelic scene in *The Psychedelic Experience*. Because the book was written by two Harvard professors and one grad student, it added an air of credibility to the 1960s nascent psychedelic movement and became a manual for how to relate to the experience of taking psychedelic drugs. The pages also contained some instructional elements, including giving the user some insight into what "set and setting" is and why it is so important.

The authors explain, "The nature of the experience depends almost entirely on set and setting. Set denotes the preparation of the individual, including his personality structure and his mood at the time. Setting is physical—the weather, the room's atmosphere; social—feelings of persons present towards one another; and cultural—prevailing views as to what is real. It is for this reason that manuals or guidebooks are necessary. Their purpose is to enable a person to understand the new realities of the expanded consciousness, to serve as road maps for new interior territories which modern science has made accessible."

That short passage gave tremendous insight and candor into the transformational power of the psychedelic experience. What it lacked, however, has become glaringly apparent as the years have gone by: a model for what to do after the journey, what we now refer to as "integration." Many of the millions of people who did LSD in the '60s didn't have much instruction for how to make the experience sustainable. They were chasing the magic that LSD can induce, but much of it was done haphazardly and without much guidance or structure. This led to the very seductive tendency to chase peak experiences.

The cycle of chasing peak experience revolves around the idea of getting high and then coming back down again. And thus, people tend to repeat that cycle over and over again, thinking that the getting high part is the actual work within the psychedelic experience. It is not. The work comes from doing your best to maximize the time spent in each psychedelic journey by taking your insights and turning them into action. This is what I mean by sustainability. The suggestions that I make in this chapter can help in making each trip a little more sustainable as opposed to an unfocused desire to grab hold of ephemeral bits of information by getting high over and over again.

In today's psychedelic landscape, there are many labels for how a journey might be structured. The most common ones are recreational use, semi-recreational use, guided use, and therapeutic use that is done under the supervision of a therapist. The good news is that all the principles in this chapter are applicable to all these ways of taking a journey.

Set: The Internal Environment

"Set" in the context of psychedelic use means to engage in a process that determines if your inner world or your mindset is in a stable place to engage in the journey. The entire process of psychedelic exploration starts by applying the concept of "set" in a way that works for you. There is no one standardized method or any one go-to workbook for how to do this. You can use the questions provided in this book, work with a psychedelic-friendly therapist, talk to an experienced psychedelic voyager, or work with a trained psychedelic guide.

On one hand, set is very easy to understand, and on the other it can be a very vague self-assessment of whether one can determine if they are a good candidate to start this process in the first place. It's tricky because it is entirely up to the individual to determine for themselves if they have a healthy set within their own mind. Only you can decide that. Sure, a trained psychedelic therapist can lead you down the road, but only you can make the final decision. This creates many problems. The well-intentioned inner hunger to discover your mind's inner workings and the very nature of reality can be so seductive that patience and discipline can often be cast aside. The wild, unhinged nature of the 1960s and its eventual collapse illustrate this. Far too many young people took LSD even though they most likely were not in the right headspace to do it in the first place. Even though that was the minority, it did create some real problems and gave way to the social narrative that psychedelic drugs can lead to psychosis or extreme behavior. The minority of users who had destabilizing experiences gave fuel to an antidrug sentiment that was already brewing.

Now, thanks to the medical application of psychedelics, which has enshrined a rigorous approach to using psychedelic drugs, we have many methods to give the new generation of psychonauts on how best to use these powerful mind-altering chemicals even in self-administered or recreational settings. It is my hope that by doing so, it will lessen the number of challenging trips and increase the overall efficacy of positive psychedelic use.

Putting sacred and personal recreational use aside for a minute and shifting focus to the psychedelic-assisted therapy model, what comes to light is the very best of the modern psychedelic renaissance's embrace of the medicalization model, data, and strong methodology on how to use these powerful psychotropic agents. This is one of the greatest achievements of the medicalized psychedelic movement. The clinically oriented process, from beginning to end, is supervised entirely by a trained professional who can help the voyager determine if they are in the right headspace to be doing this work at all and be there with them throughout the entire process. This is who we refer to as a "guide" or "psychedelic therapist."

Even before the administration of the drug happens, the screening process is designed to determine if psychedelic-assisted therapy is right for the person at this stage in their healing process. For instance, if we look at the MAPS clinical trials for treating PTSD with MDMA, the screening process that the potential participants went through was so rigorous that hundreds of applicants were turned away. The protocol for Phase 3 clinical trials, which are the last clinical trials before FDA approval, stated the following:

> Participants will be persons aged 18 or older, with a confirmed diagnosis of at least severe PTSD per the PCL-5 (PTSD Checklist for DSM-5) at Screening with symptoms present for at least 6 months. Participants would not be excluded for having more than one traumatic event or for having tried, not tolerated, or refused a selective serotonin reuptake inhibitor (SSRI) or serotonin norepinephrine reuptake inhibitor (SNRI) prescribed for PTSD. Participants with confirmed diagnosis of specific psychological and personality disorders will be excluded. Participants must be in good physical

health and without major medical disorders that could affect the safety or tolerability of MDMA.

While there are no deeper definitions of what "specific psychological and personality disorders" are in this case, it is indicative that even with severe PTSD, the participants' set must be in a place that is receptive to the combination of the drug and corresponding therapy.

Generally speaking, there are some severe psychiatric disorders and some all-around low energy states of consciousness that don't do well with psychedelic use and make for a subpar set:

- Schizophrenia: People with schizophrenia may have a preexisting vulnerability in their brain chemistry that makes them more susceptible to the disruptive effects of psychedelics.

- Bipolar 1 and 2.

- Personality disorders, such as borderline personality disorder.

- Bad attitudes: Resistant, outwardly combative, violent, and completely dismissive mindsets are all examples of attitudes that I would suggest aren't right for psychedelic use. That doesn't mean these can't change over time, but for now, hit the pause button.

This list is by no means comprehensive, and there are some who disagree with the notion that these are hard nos for taking psychedelics. In fact, the *Journal of Psychopharmacology* ran a study surveying 541 people with bipolar disorder in which two thirds of them claimed that psilocybin helped them reduce their bipolar symptoms, while the other third cited a worsening of symptoms. There are shades of gray. The research being done in reassessing the treatment of these conditions using psychedelics is promising and might have us rethink how we deal with them and the use of psychedelics; however, as a general guideline for safety and efficacy, it's wise to wait and do some more inner work before taking psychedelics if you currently suffer from any of these conditions.

For the (probably) millions of other Americans who are either considering using psychedelics or already are, the challenge for how to assess one's readiness is at a crossroads. On one hand, there is more information out there now for how to set someone up for success than ever before. Books like *The Psychedelic Explorer's Guide* by Dr. James Fadiman give good overviews on how to approach using psychedelics safely and wisely. On the other hand, the barrage of headlines that psychedelic research has gained in the treatment of mental health issues has created a huge rush for the general public to adopt using these medicines themselves without much of an understanding of the process as a whole.

In all my years of being in this movement, I've never seen curiosity at this level. More people come to me thinking that these drugs are somehow magic pills that can heal them in a single dose or that just because they want to do psychedelics in a highly intentional way, it somehow gives them a pass on having to do all the additional work that is required to create a successful outcome from using psychedelics as a healing tool. As an observer, advisor, and sometimes facilitator, I see many signs that someone isn't in the right headspace or "set" to use psychedelics at this point in time.

Firstly, because of the swell in popularity surrounding psychedelic healing, more and more first timers are interested in the method. While this is mostly a good thing, it does also lead to excited newcomers being in a huge rush to reap the potential benefits. What I look for is how they balance curiosity with desperation. If it skews too hard to the latter, then I find that as a red flag. Mental health issues, sadness, heartbreak, and the challenges of living life are all factors that may result in someone wanting to try a method for healing. Many of us have tried a myriad of approaches that haven't done much, and turning to psychedelics as a last resort is becoming more and more common—and often successful. There's nothing wrong with the "last house on the block" sentiment that many who have hit rock bottom have found ourselves in. But the intangible quality of desperation can also lead to impulsiveness and a drifting away from a careful and deliberate methodological approach in making good decisions, especially ones that can impact our health in a positive way. Coming into psychedelic healing desperate and panicked can lead to someone not allowing space for the medicine to meet them where they truly are. I advise anyone who is suffering and wants to consider psychedelics as a healing method to slow down and make sure all the boxes are checked before proceeding.

What that means in a practical sense is to make sure you have all the supplementary support mechanisms in place before moving forward. This may include a support system (friends, support group, a partner who supports this work), a psychedelic-friendly therapist, and some form of a contemplative practice like meditation or breathwork. Additionally, if you are using psychedelics to treat mental health, it's also helpful to know about the other methods that have been explored, even if they have failed to provide relief.

Moving forward in this chapter, we'll explore some questions and exploratory topics that can help paint a better picture for one's set before going into the journey.

A Checklist for Psychedelics and Mental Health

If you are at the end of the road and have tried everything else to alleviate your suffering for whatever mental health condition you have, it's natural to have an elevated impatience and want to throw yourself into the wonders of psychedelic healing. Before you do that, here are some questions you might want to ask yourself.

- Are you currently on any psychiatric medications?
- Are you isolated and alone, without a support system in place (for example, a therapist, group support, peer support, family support, etc.)?

- Are you rushing into psychedelics because of the research you've read?

- If you are suffering from a mental health condition, have you explored other methods like therapy?

- Are you lacking the complementary tools for before and after the journey, such as yoga, meditation, breathwork, etc.?

If you answered yes to any of these questions, which are contra-indicators, then it's likely that psychedelics aren't right for you at this point in time. That doesn't mean this won't always be the case, but it's essential that if you are seeking treatment for mental health using psychedelics, you view this as a holistic treatment option and not one that exists in a vacuum.

Basically, what I look for in those who are in a mental health predicament is whether or not they have an already existing holistic wellness routine to supplement the psychedelic therapy *and* a grounded set of expectations on what psychedelic healing can offer them. If these can be articulated and seem to be in place, then I feel comfortable starting the conversation with them about plotting out a psychedelic-assisted treatment protocol.

Chasing the Peak Experience

"I've been shooting in the dark too long. When something's not right, it's wrong."

—Bob Dylan

Abstract and not easily defined, a key quality (which is really a problem) that I look for in psychedelic voyagers who come to me is their ability to express balance in their desires for wanting to do a guided journey. This mainly applies to the more mystically inclined psychonaut who has previous experience and not so much the mental health scenario. Are they here for real and tangible intentions, or are they here to have yet another peak experience? This is another somewhat opaque but necessary investigation into the potential psychedelic voyager.

In other words, have they been over-using psychedelics? Terence McKenna once said, "What we drug people have that others do not is repetition." Terence was a once-in-a-generation thinker whose foundation was so strong that he could go back time and time again into the DMT netherworlds without much detriment. His model for becoming a "self-initiated" mystic—who also stated the best way to use psilocybin mushrooms is to take five grams in the dark alone—wasn't reckless coming from him. But in today's psychedelic world, where we are trying to disseminate a more cautious and slow burn approach, it's also not recommended.

Or when you hear the story of Richard Alpert taking LSD every weekend in the gatehouse at Millbrook for the better part of a year, you tend to forget that he had the pedigree of a Harvard researcher trying to break through the confounding realization that you have to "come down." About six months after the Millbrook gatehouse self-induced experiments, he solved the predicament when he met Neem Karoli Baba and was given a new map of consciousness. The end result was that he didn't stop using psychedelics, but he did so with far less frequency and without the topsy-turvy side effect of coming up and down over and over again. That's because he saw he was chasing peak experiences and wasn't looking at the use of psychedelics as a holistic part of an overall spiritual quest. He was using them in a vacuum. After he fully morphed into Ram Dass, it's safe to say that his entire life was one big peak experience of love, compassion, and the endless quest to spread the teachings of his guru through action.

Bottom line, psychedelic drugs are best used infrequently and with a plan that is built around extracting the most you can possibly get out of each and every single trip.

Recreational Versus Assisted Use

The term "recreational use" conjures up images of so many pop culture clichés, like Burners rolling on MDMA or Deadheads tripping and spinning to the magical adventure of Jerry's guitar riffs. In today's psychedelic world, I use the term "recreational use" to mean anything other than formal psychedelic-assisted therapy. It is not a derogatory term that implies flippant and careless uses of these compounds; it is an expansive menu of applications that may include spiritual growth, connection with nature, connection with a romantic partner, community building, and all-around transcendental exploration. We have been gifted with so much research and data that in turn has given even the recreational user a blueprint for how best to go on a psychedelic journey. Because of that, it's important to make the distinction that recreational use does not necessarily mean dangerous or careless.

> **Recreational use:** Acid heads at a Dead show or MDMA
> users at Burning Man are perhaps the most clichéd (but
> accurate) depictions of recreational use. Since I am a product
> of countless amounts of LSD trips at Grateful Dead concerts,
> I can't denounce this way of taking psychedelics. However, I
> do wish I had been given better information all of those
> years ago. Recreational use is here to stay, and the most
> effective way to keep those users as safe as possible is through
> education and harm reduction. Even the most reckless
> recreational user can be dealt a better hand if they apply the
> principles of set and setting, and perhaps pause and reflect in
> hopes of not making a poor decision.

> **Semi-recreational use:** This might look like gathering with
> friends to create a container that is spiritually focused, rooted
> in intention setting, and has a formal application of set
> and setting that can be done as a way of creating a built-in
> support system. The experienced psychonaut can help make
> sure that the session and the friends that are gathered are

prepared not just for their own sakes but for others should the need arise.

Guided use: The first thing that comes to mind for me in this category is taking psychedelics under the supervision of a shaman, a curandera, or a trained psychedelic guide. For example, going on an Ayahuasca retreat in Peru will be structured, safe, and ceremonial but might not contain any written set and setting exercises or intention setting. Even in that situation, you can add to the ceremony by doing your own self-guided preparation work and working with an integration coach afterward.

Therapeutic use: Most commonly referred to as psychedelic-assisted therapy and what is most commonly found in the medicalized model. Any good psychedelic-assisted therapist will do a rigorous amount of pre-journey intention setting, psychosocial explorations to ensure readiness, and medical screening to make sure the voyager will react to the medicine well. The therapist will be in the room with you at all times helping you piece together what is happening during the session and most of all to keep you safe.

There are so many resources available at the touch of a button (thanks Google) that I think are prudent to dive into before going on your first psychedelic voyage or even your twentieth. It makes me passionate about the idea that it's better to provide solid prep, intention, and integration models before having a peak experience than it is to encourage the sudden repetition of the peak experience itself.

Profit-driven psychedelic enterprises are also partially to blame for the rotating door, amusement park model of taking psychedelic drugs. Much of the overuse of psychedelics is the result of aggressive psychedelic facilitators or retreat owners who make a fair sum of money guiding people on their vision quests—essentially psychedelic Disneylands. Their marketing can come across like an astral swashbuckling hero's journey that you simply can't miss—and if you do, you are not actualizing your full potential! "Don't miss out on this once-in-a-lifetime opportunity to reveal your connection in the multiverse!"

The providers I gravitate toward the most, and the ones I recommend, are the ones who are hard to find, the ones who don't market themselves or have any self-styled labels around their names that turn them into cartoon characters of the psychedelic movement. These providers are humble, aren't phony-holy, and are compassionate. They warn you just as much about the shadow as they do the light. They make no illusions that this is difficult work and that you must be ready on all fronts before voyaging.

Chasing a peak experience in psychedelics is no different than in any other medium. That revelation from an experience can burn so bright that you can't help but want to do it again and again. That's natural to an extent. We all want to reexperience pleasurable moments in our lives. What makes psychedelics different is that each experience you have is totally different from the last, and the law of diminishing returns applies. You can never experience the same "aha moment" again.

Because each peak psychedelic experience sheds light on a different part of your overall human makeup, it's best to dive deep into what that singular experience did for you and how it can help improve your life. It's not that multiple sessions can't provide constructive excavation, but if you aren't careful and just set out on blind repetition, things can start to get a little cluttered and far too abstract—a million little pieces in the ether that need piecing back together again. Either that or you become too familiar with the far-off landscapes and start using the drugs as escapist tools. Either way, one of the great rewards that the modern psychedelic movement has brought us are rigid methodologies for how best to use our time on psychedelics. It all begins with intention: Why do you want to do this in the first place?

Intentions

For whatever reason you find yourself considering the use of psychedelics, it starts with the setting of an intention. The why. Being merely curious isn't enough for me. Sentiments like, "Oh, I just want to see what these drugs are about. I've read so much about them that I want to see for myself, but I really have no idea what they can do for me," are potentially dangerous and create a space for the unpredictable potential of these drugs to overwhelm the person. Being clear on the intentions you want to bring into your ceremony is a good sign that your "set" is off to a good start.

Therefore, it's really important that you do your best to verbalize your intentions with either a trained psychedelic-assisted therapist if you are using them for mental health reasons or a very experienced guide if you are considering them for something else. If you are going solo, write down your answers to the questions I posed in chapter 2.

Our issues, stories, emotional damage, and trauma are usually the most common seeds for bringing intentions to the light. I like to encourage people to at least be open to the idea that your issues are just one part of you and do not have to control your every waking moment. Even if they do right now, just be open to the idea that they don't later. Once you are able to have a vision that is beyond the constraints of the physical world, then you are able to see that your depression, anxiety, or trauma just is. It's neither good nor bad, it just is. It may be painful, valid, and overwhelming, but if you refrain from applying labels to the struggles of your humanity, it can allow space for them to not keep a hold of you. It doesn't mean that experiencing prolonged unordinary states of consciousness like the one psychedelics can offer is a magic bullet that will instantly free you from suffering, but it does mean that a potential new perspective can be offered that can lead you to a long-term healing process that you hadn't been able to see prior.

Nonordinary States of Consciousness

Exploring a reality that is different than our waking reality is the essence of why I continue to value the psychedelic experience as a tool for continued growth and introspection. Our ordinary waking states of consciousness can, at times, keep us restrained and locked into a narrow view of our potential and our view of the world. When our frequencies are expanded to allow different points of view, both mystical and pragmatic, it's as if another road suddenly appears, one that had been there all along but was clouded by self-limiting belief systems, fears, and old ideas.

With the exception of extreme religious experiences, Western culture has distanced itself over the years from nonordinary states of consciousness. Dualistic Christian traditions like the Pentecostal Church encourage their members to be overtaken by the presence of the Lord by speaking in tongues or let their body get overwhelmed by rapid seizure-like movements that indicate they are in the presence of spirit. But these external practices don't do much for changing how people might experience themselves. In fact it perpetuates the idea that God is somehow separate from us, that God is indeed an external anthropomorphic being that we must be subservient to.

In the essential book *Autobiography of a Yogi*, Paramahansa Yogananda recalls a meditation session early on in his transformation where his guru was present and recognized his struggle with control. "He struck gently on my chest above my heart. My body became immovably rooted; breath was drawn out of my lungs as if by some huge magnet. Soul and mind instantly lost their physical bondage, and streamed out like a fluid piercing light from every pore. The flesh was as though dead, yet in my intense awareness I knew that never before had I been fully alive. My sense of identity was no longer narrowly confined to a body, but embraced the circumambient atoms . . . My ordinary frontal vision was now changed to a vast spherical sight, simultaneously all-perceptive."

Typically, in the modern world, if one is to say that they communed with an otherworldly state of being that brought them peace, contentedness, and a change in perception, they may be quickly labeled "weird" or even possibly schizophrenic, whereas the ancient sages of India would make no issue of encouraging yogis to jump around from one plane of existence to the other. That's just daily life to them.

The scientific method has certainly evolved over the last century to include more esoteric points of view around the nature of reality, but it is still based in testing and data. Daniel J. Siegel, a Western doctor whom I love and whose books I recommend, says in his fascinating book on the human need for connection called *IntraConnected*, "Science is a term we use to generally denote a rigorous way humans observe patterns in the world and create hypotheses about what that world is like. In Western science, we test those ideas with experimental paradigms to challenge our viewpoints and confirm, or disprove, our proposals on the nature of nature; on the way reality functions."

In the vast amounts of recent psychedelic research, there have been many attempts to try to define the mystical experience with tools like the Mystical Experience Questionnaire (MEQ), a self-report used in lab studies of psychedelics to measure mystical-type experiences. But from where I sit (and based on my experience), mysticism and nonordinary states of consciousness are best left partially undefinable. There is a certain noetic quality that can't be categorized, explained, or put into a data set. This is unmistakably true, and when people I encounter have a problem with this, I ask them why they think their dreams are all that different from the rest of their waking reality. Why are you so quick to dismiss dreams as just ramblings of your subconscious?

I say all this because if you go into psychedelic work thinking that your cognitive mind will lead the conversation in terms of getting relief or insights of your intentions, then you will be left with a gap in understanding what truly happened during your experience.

When it comes time to begin the process of writing one's intentions down, I encourage the user to become familiar with the idea that those intentions won't necessarily be met with linear verbal responses from the medicine. The medicine speaks to you in a way that sometimes has no language at all. It may be energetic or based on feelings that you can't quite put into words. An example of that may be writing down the intention "I want to learn how to address my anger in a healthy way and not be so explosive." Now, if you are expecting the medicine to tell you in words how you might accomplish this, you may end up even more confused than when you began. Instead, the medicine can lead you to a place where you are able to sense your emotional imbalance that lies within your behaviors, impulses, relationships, or childhood memories in a way that will have you rethink acting on your anger before it becomes damaging. These are important concepts to keep in mind before you set forth on plotting out your intentions in whatever form your guide or therapist has in place.

The following questions are my blueprint for how you can arrive at establishing your intentions for your psychedelic journey. They come from the workbook I have used with over two hundred voyagers that I have guided, and they have been the seeds for other guides to build upon to create their own framework for guiding those in need.

By doing your best to create a written blueprint for your psychedelic journey, you will create a cosmic line in the sand that lets the medicine, your guide, and spirit know that you are ready to face whatever comes up head-on. There's something very cathartic in actually writing things down. It adds a level of depth to it. Whereas when we say things out loud, they tend to come and go. Speech can be fleeting, but the written word remains. It's with this type of vulnerability and honesty that you can start shifting into the place of receptivity.

Intentions, Set, and Discovery Questions

> "The goal is to discover who you really
> are, not who you think you are."
>
> —Ram Dass

1. Who do you think you are at this stage of your life? Do you feel good about who that person is?

2. Who do you want to become in this lifetime (if different than the above answer)?

3. What role do you see psychedelics playing in this discovery?

4. What other methods (i.e., yoga, meditation, therapy, breathwork) do you currently practice that aid in your healing? If there are none, please talk about one or two that you'd like to weave into your practice. Remember, psychedelics are not a magic pill. They don't prohibit you from doing the work after the journey. Having additional methods to solidify your psychedelic discoveries is essential.

5. Do you fear taking a psychedelic substance, and what are the roots of these fears?

6. What is it you fear will happen to you?

7. Do you fear that you will confront something that may not be pleasant? Memories? Somatic recall? Why would it be unpleasant?

8. What has happened in your past that makes you fearful of reliving it? This may include past behaviors, traumas, etc.

9. Are you fearful of achieving success in the present or future?

10. Are you ready to let go of any or all of these fears?

11. Are you ready to accept that these fears, while valid, are ultimately holding you back from your healing?

12. Write out your vision for a fear-free psychedelic journey and what that looks like to you.

13. Describe your current spiritual condition. Do you feel connected to spirit? Do you have a spiritual practice? If so, what does that look like? If not, describe something that you'd like to explore.

14. Describe your sexual health. Do you feel in touch with your body and the exchange of intimacy? If you are uncomfortable expressing this in words, internalize it. Sexual health and physical balance are a key part of overall wellness and the releasing of trauma.

15. Describe and assess your physical health. Do you exercise? Do you eat well?

16. Describe and assess your personal "set." Do you feel emotionally stable? Secure? Well balanced? Are you ready to take the journey, and do you feel that it's the right time? Be candid about any potential red flags and what you can do to alleviate them.

17. What brought you to make the decision of undergoing a healing/therapeutically based psychedelic journey?

18. Are you looking to heal or grow spiritually?

19. What is it you want to heal? Be specific in regards to traumas, behaviors, etc. Write it out.

20. If you are looking to grow spiritually or otherwise, write down what that looks like. What is your definition of a spiritual connection? What other areas do you want to grow in?

21. Now, write your intentions as they arise. Try to listen to the voice that comes from your soul and not your mind. Use this space to add goals for this psychedelic session. Keep your intentions down to three or four things/areas/ categories that you would like to focus on during the upcoming journey. Remember, unraveling your entire life in one journey probably won't happen. It's useful to be specific about what's coming up for you at this moment in time.

To make it abundantly clear, it is my belief that the experience while on psychedelic drugs is not the work in and of itself. It's the fertilization stage that creates the embryo for the real work that comes after. The trip itself is anywhere from a four- to twelve-hour journey that may reveal what your ultimate destination is, which is why knowing that destination is necessary. The psychedelic journey and its final destination are two very distinct places.

Now that we've covered some of the initial planning questions and topics that are wise to consider before embarking on psychedelic work, I want to point out once again that the trip itself will show you aspects of your inner workings that may be life-changing, but what you do with that information upload afterward is where the real work begins. Any lasting impact you hope to gain after embarking on a psychedelic journey becomes truly meaningful only when you put it into practice. This is what we refer to as "integration." But before that happens, it's important to assess the setting. Where you are going to have the experience is vital for success.

Setting: The External Environment

As I've mentioned before, I grew up taking LSD in the traveling circus that was the caravan that followed Grateful Dead around the country. In today's psychedelic world, many would say that is not a healthy "setting" in which to do psychedelic drugs.

"Setting" is the environment you surround yourself with that will act as the container for your psychedelic experience. For the most part, it's true that doing powerful psychedelics like LSD in festival or concert environments surrounded by tens of thousands of people, like a Grateful Dead show, aren't recommended. While communities like Deadheads or Burners do offer a safety net of sorts, it is recommended that you treat your physical environment with as much care and attention as you do determining your mindset going into a psychedelic experience.

If you are doing a journey in your home, make sure you have a quiet room that won't be disturbed by outside noise, pets, electronic devices, and possibly your roommates. I can tell you from experience that even the slightest outside noise can set your journey off in an unwelcome direction. In the '90s, I once took a fairly large amount of LSD at my home and accidentally left the answering machine on. In the middle of the trip, the phone rang, and my mother left a voice mail that was audible throughout the entire house and into the LSD session. Needless to say the contents of that voice mail set my journey off into a direction I did not want to go down, and I spent the next several hours trying to steer myself in another direction. Don't make the same mistake.

Making your room ceremonial, sacred, and special is also strongly advised. I believe with all my heart that the psychedelic experience is mystical in nature and that your physical environment should reflect that. This may include setting up an altar with religious or spiritual artifacts that are important to you or having objects that resonate strongly with your life. This doesn't have to reflect a religious offering per se, just as long as it feels sacred to you. Adding flowers is also recommended. Having something alive and colorful in proximity can add so much depth to your experience.

The next topic is something I could write an entire chapter on, and that's music. The music you choose for your psychedelic experience is perhaps the most important physical choice you can make for your journey. I can't state how important this is. Music can take you down pathways and little nooks and crannies within your subconscious that you otherwise might not be able to access. Melodies and rhythms become such a vital part of your energetic experience, so choose wisely. The general rule of thumb is that you select music that has no lyrics, or at least no English lyrics. Look, I grew up taking copious amounts of LSD and listening to the Grateful Dead, Pink Floyd, and Yes, but I admit that the lyrical content of those bands will also affect your emotional resonance. They will steer you in a very specific direction. It's wise to start with ambient world music, tribal music, or even classical music. If you don't know where to start, you'll be pleasantly surprised to know that there are many psychedelic journey playlists on Spotify. Countless psychonauts have put together wonderfully thoughtful playlists for you to start. And to take it a step further, there are even artists, like East Forest and Jon Hopkins, who have made entire albums for assisting the psychedelic experience. *IN: A Soundtrack for the Psychedelic Practitioner* by East Forest is a beautifully soulful and introspective album that is worthy of your first two hours of any journey. However, once you have some insight into the natural rhythms of the psychedelic landscape, I recommend that you start creating your own playlists, being sensitive to the come up, the peak, and the comedown.

Everything I've mentioned here should also apply to any medicine work you might do in a clinical or medical setting. As mentioned, one of my biggest gripes with the medicalization of psychedelics is that it's become far too sterile. There is no good reason why any psychedelic experience needs to be done in a sterile white room with no love or care put into it. If you happen to find yourself in a situation like this, please ask your provider if some changes can be made to the physical environment that can make you feel more at ease, comfortable, and prone to increase mystical results. Push back if they say no. This is your journey to create, and the therapist in the room should be there to keep you safe and help you accomplish what you need, but they are not there to dictate how the experience should go.

Integration: Making for a More Sustainable Experience

Integration discussions are thankfully coming into practice in this new psychedelic renaissance we find ourselves in; however, there is no one formal methodology or protocol that is used or should be used. My aim here is to provide one option, a protocol, that you can use to make the transformation you experienced in your psychedelic experience long-lasting, practical, and sustainable. The extreme cycles of coming up and down no longer have to be part of the psychedelic experience. Nor do the fleeting, ephemeral little glimpses of peering into the veil of mystery need to be relegated to the esoteric. They too can be translated into meaningful metaphors that you can apply to your daily life. What belief systems you subscribe to and what type of life you've made for yourself also don't matter. If you are a spiritual person, a biohacker, a career person, an artist, or a college dropout, it doesn't matter in the eyes of God. What does matter is that you take ownership of your individual sovereignty and do what it takes to live your most authentic life that is most appropriate for your path.

You may still be asking the question, "What is integration exactly?"

When writing the outline for this book, I was discussing with my partner Heather, a licensed therapist who also works in the space, my many musings around integration. As someone who helps others achieve their psychedelic goals, I put so much emphasis on integration and why it's so important. I can't stress enough that putting all this effort into this experience is nothing if it's not long-lasting. After much discussion, she replied, "SUSTAINABILITY! That's it, that's what you've always been talking about. It's the third S. Set, setting, and sustainability." Indeed, I couldn't be more grateful for her push in helping me simplify this concept into something that is easily digestible and even makes for a good bumper sticker.

In its simplest form, integration means you engage in a process that assigns meaning to your psychedelic experience. That process can be self-guided, or it can be supervised by a psychedelic-friendly therapist or integration coach. The primary reason this is so important is that, for decades, many psychedelic drug users found it so difficult to come back from those altered states to deliver meaningful insights into what occurred. The culture itself lacked any real instructions for how one might do this, and it seemed that only a select few were able to really translate the psychedelic experience into words that others could relate to. Terence McKenna, Ram Dass, Stan Grof, and Timothy Leary come to mind. But millions of hippie kids were taking loads of LSD during the 1960s and found themselves dreaming of a new world full of love, tolerance, and a universal sense of equanimity. Problem is, it didn't work out as well as planned.

Perhaps because of that, it is my intention that everything you find in this section is intended to be practical. It is designed to maximize the amount of self-love in your life and minimize the amount of self-loathing and other fear-based defense mechanisms. It is also designed to offer some self-analytical tools for you to map out your consciousness in a way that is both pragmatic and mystical—a "mind map" if you will. Any skilled psychonaut will tell you that their consciousness is forever altered as a result of the psychedelic experience, and I encourage you to document that as best as you can.

My suggestion is that you take the realizations you had from your journey, both positive and challenging, and hold them in equal value. You cannot ignore or run away from the negative parts of your humanity. They are part of you, for better or for worse. I am merely suggesting that with the self-reflection that comes after a psychedelic journey, you can get to the point where you know with absolute conviction that they no longer serve you.

Is your story of having a traumatic childhood the primary narrative that's guided you into despair and struggle? Do you have such a close relationship with it that it's affected your relationships, your work, and your ability to choose love over destruction? Perhaps you come from a long lineage of alcoholics who gave you a false narrative that abuse and neglect are the norm for the family unit. Or maybe you were never able to find your own footing in life, and pleasure-seeking mechanisms became your go-to for being alive. Drug, food, or sex addiction and the overstimulation of dopamine became so comforting that you found you couldn't live without it.

Whatever your case may be, I empathize with it greatly and know firsthand that real change can be slow going. I have also noticed in my years within various groups and spiritual healing circles that there can be a tendency to hang on to our traumatic pasts and limiting belief systems like badges of honor. There's a certain comfort in hanging on to our "stuckness." I encourage us all to take a look at that paradigm and truly imagine what it would be like to be free from suffering.

A successful psychonaut must be open to the idea that their traumas, while painful, can be shifted to a place in which they no longer have to govern your emotional well-being. The goal is that under the right set and setting and with a rigorous integration protocol, a well-planned psychedelic session will get you to the point of not having to hang on to your suffering and its accompanying stories so tightly.

Set, Setting, and Sustainability: A Post-Journey Road Map for Long-Term Integration Success

"Integration, like so many things in the beautifully fickle
psychedelic space, often laughs in our face when we
try to define it, or God forbid standardize it."

—Jack Kornfield

Again, before you begin your journey, I recommend that you work alongside a trained guide or a psychedelic-friendly therapist who can support you along the way. You might get triggered from having to recall challenging parts of your experience, and it's only natural to want to run away from that. Having a trained professional with you can help reinforce safety and give you tips for how to regulate the unraveling of what might have been a very complex matrix of autobiographical realizations.

In the following sections, I offer some preliminary steps and suggestions that I've found to be necessary for grounding and tapping into states that bring joy or relaxation and support a state of remembering. If you are an experienced psychonaut, then you can use these suggestions as a self-guided framework for your continued growth and unfolding.

Contemplative Practices

After any psychedelic experience, it's important that you continue to practice any method, technique, or discipline that is considered a contemplative practice. As discussed in chapter 2, the default mode network (DMN) works incredibly hard to discount nonordinary states of consciousness experiences by limiting our perception of reality and throwing us back into everyday life. The seven to ten days after a journey are the sweet spots where you can remember, document, and integrate the big changes you want to take away from your experience. This can be greatly helped by making sure you do your method of choice during that time frame.

To make the point, an extreme example of what not to do would be to do a psychedelic journey on Sunday and then go back to work on Monday. This defeats the whole purpose and wouldn't serve you. Contemplative practices like meditation, yoga, and breathwork are effective tools to use after a psychedelic journey because they can help you tap back into that state of being you experienced during your journey. They can help you slow the waking state activity of your mind and aid you in becoming more reflective of what just transpired. Most people who have used psychedelics successfully take some time after their journey, maybe two to three days, to sit quietly and reflect before jumping back into their day-to-day lives. I'd go so far as to say that it's a requirement that you build in and plan this after-journey time buffer before you even take the journey. If you don't have the time, then it's not the right time.

Things You Love to Do/Enriching Hobbies

In some ways, the things you love to do can also be considered contemplative practices. You'll hear many musicians talk about being in a "flow state" when they get lost in their instrument. Most of us have a hobby that brought us joy in the past, but because of our busy life it has been put on the back burner. Are you a fledgling guitarist or painter who rarely finds the time to spend on it? Do you write poems or short stories but get hung up on the idea that no one will read them, so why bother? Sentiments like these are ideal to revisit after your psychedelic experience. Hobbies like these are for yourself and your own personal satisfaction. Even if you're not very good, picking up the guitar after a journey can no doubt help you relax and enjoy your newfound sense of expansiveness. Play like no one is listening, dance like no one is watching, sing like you are a rock star. You may find that you might not only commit to finding more time for these hobbies but you may actually improve at them thanks to your psychedelic experience.

Be kind to yourself and know that even if your psychedelic experience was challenging, there are beneficial takeaways that can improve your life. Doing any of the aforementioned practices or hobbies are ways to help you slow down and get closer to the realizations you experienced during your journey.

Pre-Integration Practical Suggestions

In the days following a psychedelic journey, you might find that many of the realizations you had during the journey start to fade away and become almost dreamlike. This is normal and to be expected; however, it can also be combated by following some basic guidelines to help you integrate your experience.

- If you are working with a guide during the session, relay any realizations while they are happening. Say them out loud so your guide can write them down.

- Upon conclusion of your journey, journal or voice-memo any realizations you had during the journey. I offer some questions and writing prompts in the next section. Pay attention to how they relate to your life and emotional intelligence.

- Do not go immediately back to your daily routine the day after a journey (i.e., work, school, etc.). Take the day after to journal, reflect, and bring into focus anything that happened during the journey that was a part of you and not a foreign visitor purely influenced by the drug.

- The seven days post-journey are the most important. These seven days are when your brain is the most malleable and when it is most possible to offset the function of the default mode network. It's not a perfect science or practice, but meditation, sharing with others, and journaling can help.

- It's essential that you meditate on the three or four biggest takeaways from the journey for seven days following the journey. Write these down and turn them into mantras that can be focused on during your meditation practice. The repetition while in meditation acts as a way to slow your thinking mind and create the possibility of forming new neuronal networks.

The Five Stages of Integration

The primary goal is to turn insight into action. Lofty and ephemeral insights are all fine and well but don't mean much unless we turn them into actual actions that can benefit our lives on a daily basis. These five states are some loose suggestions for how to make that happen.

1. **Receiving and remembering:** Work with your guide and intuition to receive the downloads that come to you during the journey. Pay special attention to the subtle shifts and messages and, of course, to the major downloads. Do whatever you can to remember them: say them out loud to your guide or write them down after. Remember, they might not come in the form of words and might be just a feeling or an energetic shift.

2. **Processing the journey:** Process your journey through meditation, discussion, and bringing it into your traditional therapeutic relationship (if applicable). This is how you begin the process of assigning meaning to your experience.

3. **Being aware of old habits and making connections for new ones:** After completing the following integration

questions, you should have more awareness of how your old habits and belief systems have manifested in your life. Allow space for new connections that morph into new behaviors.

4. **Sharing with others:** Share your experience with friends, romantic partners, or in an integration circle. Community and outward expression help externalize the ephemeral.

5. **Into action—micro habits:** Take your main downloads and turn them into action steps. This is the primary method for sustainability. How can we make these experiences last? Why is that important?

Integration Questions

To help combat the "fading away" of your journey's primary downloads, writing about your journey can help solidify your experience. Here are some questions and prompts to consider after your journey so you have a record of your trip. This record will be useful when you want to revisit the details of your journey days, months, or years in the future.

1. What substance did you take, and what was the dosage?

2. Describe the set and setting for your journey. Did you use a guide, or did you journey with a friend or on your own?

3. Do you feel like you stayed true to the intentions you stated prior to your journey?

4. Isolate one of your main intentions for the session and describe how it manifested during the trip.

5. Describe what your relationship with your intentions is like now. Do they still feel relevant? If one of your intentions was healing the pain of your past, for example, describe how you feel about that pain now that you've looked at it during a session. Do you feel less

attached to the idea that the pain needs to cause you continued suffering? (This could be trauma inflicted by others, trauma inflicted by yourself, death and dying issues, tumultuous relationships, addiction behaviors, etc.)

6. Can you imagine a life free from the bondage of the past?

7. If one of your intentions or journey downloads was about your evolution into your future self, do you feel comfortable and at ease with the person you are becoming? Be honest about where you are and the person you see in the "mirror."

8. Describe any pleasure you experienced during the trip. Was it physical, sensual, spiritual, or emotional?

9. If you were using the psychedelic session to gain more clarity around what you want to be doing with your time, do you feel that you gained more insight into that? Do you feel that you are putting your energy into the right places?

10. Describe what you want to be doing in life now that the journey is over. Did this change much from when you answered the same question before the journey?

11. Try to isolate the big events that happened during the trip. Describe the three most important moments.

12. Take those three most important realizations and try to explain why they are important to your life on a daily basis.

13. Describe your relationship with the world around you. Do you feel at peace with your surroundings, your job, your home life, family life, and social life?

14. Describe your view of a spiritual connection now that you have completed a session. Did it change as a result of the trip?

15. If you used MDMA, how does your body feel post-session? Did you take the re-uptake supplements?

16. If you used mushrooms, LSD, or DMT and the trip was highly visual, try to describe what those visions were like.

17. Did those visions feel completely random or part of a bigger message?

18. Now that you've done some work using psychedelics as a method, describe how you see psychedelics playing an ongoing role in your life.

19. As a result of these questions and your overall perception, write down three things you can do differently in your life starting today.

20. Write any general concerns, feelings, realizations, or thoughts you have about the session you experienced. After you've completed these twenty questions, use this space for seven additional days after the journey to make note of what's evolved over the course of time. Meditate on your answers.

The Jack Kornfield quote that began this section says specifically that we should never "god forbid standardize" the integration process. I couldn't agree with that more, and my suggestions above are intended to provide you with a blueprint of sorts that you can personalize and adapt in ways that work best for you. There is no one way to do integration at all, just so long as you're doing it. Finding methods and techniques that speak to you are what's most important.

When it comes to set and setting, however, these suggestions are a little more firm in the reality of how they are applied. Nearly every mistake I've seen happen in the world of psychedelics has to do with poor applications of basic set and setting principles. That and impure drugs are at the root cause of when psychedelics go horribly wrong. I've mentioned it many times in this book, but again, not everyone is suited for the psychedelic experience at any given moment. Hopefully my suggestions can shed some light on whether this is the right path for you at this stage in life, and if it's not, that's okay. Be patient and prudent. There is no rush. Use every educational resource at your disposal to access the best path forward for your own inner work. You'll be glad you did in the end.

11

The Legal Situation

Balancing Access and Commercialization

"If the words 'life, liberty, and the pursuit of happiness' don't include
the right to experiment with your own consciousness, then the
Declaration of Independence isn't worth the hemp it was written on."

—Terence McKenna

We have entered a brave new world of psychedelic research and
its associated culture. Experiences, both from the individual
and within the scientific community, have created a pool of data so
extraordinary that I would not have guessed the advancement that
we are seeing today would have been possible a mere fifteen years ago.
Things are moving at lightning speed and are forcing the discussion
of how these medicines are to be used legally in nearly every Western
country across the globe. I said "Western" intentionally. Some countries elsewhere in the world have laws on the books that enact the

death sentence for possession of any recreational drug, period. That is an entirely different story and topic for another time.

Positions on the legality of psychedelic drugs in the US differ within the therapeutic community as much as they do outside of it. Some believe that the legal use of psychedelic drugs should be limited to administration only under the care of a licensed therapist, while others believe that complete recreational use should be granted to those over a certain age. I fall somewhere in the middle and, quite frankly, often contradict myself—so often in fact that many of my podcast listeners have called me out by writing me letters that say, "I thought you were all about cognitive liberty? Why are you ranting about the failure of take-home ketamine use?" I'll do my best to explain and let you know that I am sorting out my position in real time. It's a work in progress.

First, I believe in cognitive liberty—that we must be granted the right to change our own consciousness as we see fit. The very nature of consciousness is nonlinear, eternal, and infinite. It cannot be categorized or suggested that we must only interpret it through a small box that we call "reality." It's an ever-swirling, mysterious, and disembodied part of the multiverse that is dependent on human exploration via any modality that is available. Therefore, adults over the age of twenty-one should have access to safe, chemically pure, and ethically sourced psychedelic medicines just as they do alcohol or tobacco. However, I don't believe it should be a free-for-all. I am not positive that any adult should be able to walk into a headshop and buy a liquid vial of LSD that has one thousand hits in it.

Unequivocally, I firmly believe that adults should be given the power to experience their own divinity, which allows them to feel the way they want and seek methods for spiritual and cognitive growth that may incorporate the use of psychedelics. But pushing the limits of psycho-spiritual mind and soul exploration is not for the faint of heart. Psychedelics simply aren't built to suit every type of person. Mechanisms must be put in place that don't allow teenagers, for instance, to be able to buy unlimited quantities of MDMA just because they obtained a fake ID, and prevent those who are suffering from untreated mental illness to get their hands on LSD and spiral into further oblivion. This would be disastrous for the greater good. ER doctors and nurses and police, for instance, have very little sensitivity training for how to deal with someone on large amounts of psychedelics.

The specifics of how this would work involve honest discussions and collaborations between psychedelic scientists, advocates, and policy makers. The issues here are so nuanced that they could make for another book and obviously require a great amount of discussion and cooperation with all parties involved. Also, I have no answer for any of the mechanisms that I think should be put into place. I am not a policy maker and quite frankly get overwhelmed at the complexity of installing some sort of regulatory system that would need to govern safe access to psychedelics. I'll be the first to admit that even with access to unadulterated psychedelics, our society is not equipped to handle the fragile nature of someone who has a destabilizing psychedelic experience, let alone the possible masses. Therefore, I find myself contradicting myself often. On one hand, I believe in a swift end to the drug war and I think all drugs should be decriminalized, and on the other, I believe that it's naïve to think that every adult should have unlimited access to powerful consciousness-changing drugs. I encourage everyone who is a part of this community to brainstorm ideas to generate a path forward that makes sense for all parties involved, ranging from psychonauts to law enforcement.

The Failure of the War on Drugs

We live in a world that says some drugs are okay but others are not, a world that has created a War on Drugs that has fueled a global enterprise ranging from the jungles of Colombia to the streets of Compton—all of which have elements of corruption. On June 9, 2021, the Drug Policy Alliance (DPA) and the American Civil Liberties Union (ACLU) released a new poll indicating that a large majority of Americans have concluded that the War on Drugs has failed.

Unraveling the history of the War on Drugs and its three primary architects—Harry J. Anslinger, Richard Nixon, and Ronald Reagan—you will find that all three of these men helped create some of the most disastrous and blatantly racist examples of public policy in the twentieth century. From 1930 to 1962, Harry Anslinger was a significant figure in America's crusade against recreational drugs, most notably as the first commissioner of the Federal Bureau of Narcotics (FBN), a precursor to the Drug Enforcement Administration (DEA).

Cannabis had been around in the States for quite some time prior to the 1930s, but its industrialized cousin species, hemp, was more popular. Hemp was used for the manufacturing of common goods like rope and paper, while the actual smoking of the cannabis sativa plant was done quietly, without much fanfare, throughout a few segments of the population. It was part of the American agricultural and intoxicant fabric, but use prior to the 1960s certainly wasn't as common as it is now. Even so, it was never thought of as a public threat or health concern until Anslinger came along and literally made up stories that demonized the ancient plant. Anslinger was instrumental in advocating for and implementing laws that criminalized and regulated many narcotics, including cannabis. Why, you may ask? He didn't like the people who smoked it, and his level of hatred is what fueled what was known as the "reefer madness" sensation.

In the '30s, when a wave of Central Americans and Mexicans started to immigrate into the US, the environment was ripe for another round of classic American xenophobia. Cannabis was used safely and harmlessly by many Mexican workers, which only gave Anslinger more ammunition against already marginalized communities. He even changed the name of cannabis to the far more exotic and incorrect word "marijuana." The propaganda worked: it led to the passage of the Marihuana Tax Act of 1937, which effectively criminalized the possession and sale of cannabis at a federal level.

Under Anslinger's leadership, the FBN aggressively pursued campaigns against drug use and the people who used them. The "reefer madness" era propagated sensationalized narratives about the dangers of marijuana, associating its use with violence, insanity, and moral degradation. Do yourself a favor and watch the film of the same name. It's purely comedic today, but in the 1930s, it was anything but. This was how the use of cannabis was portrayed in the media of the time.

Anslinger's efforts were deeply rooted in racial biases and can be summed up by the following quote: "There are 100,000 total marijuana smokers in the US, and most are Negroes, Hispanics, Filipinos, and entertainers. Their Satanic music, jazz, and swing result from marijuana usage. This marijuana causes white women to seek sexual relations with Negroes, entertainers, and any others." That's about all you have to know about Harry Anslinger and the work he did. There's not much more you can say about that.

His tenure as the head of the FBN was marked by a relentless pursuit of strict drug policies, advocating for stringent penalties and criminalization of drug offenses, which created the first modern iteration of the War on Drugs. The anti-drug propaganda through media campaigns and public speeches shaped public perception and contributed to the stigmatization of drug users in ways we still see today.

After Prohibition ended on December 5, 1933, the two primary recreational intoxicants on the American stage were alcohol and tobacco. This went on for decades until the '60s rolled around and introduced an even more confounding problem for the Nixon administration. Many of the people who were using cannabis and some of the newer drugs on the scene, like LSD, were white. Middle-class white kids became fixtures of the anti–Vietnam War movement and formed what we now refer to as the "counterculture." Up until this point it was pretty easy for anti-drug politicians to pinpoint and attack certain populations that were using illegal drugs. Black people and Mexicans were easy targets, and finding ways to keep their communities in peril was the primary mission. When middle-class white kids started using drugs, it added a new ideological form of discrimination not really seen before in the mainstream.

Once again, we saw drugs being used by people that the establishment didn't like. Kids burning draft cards were taking LSD, so all the research in the world related to legitimate psychedelic use didn't mean a thing. It was the first to go. It became illegal in 1966 and a Schedule 1 drug in 1968, which all but made it impossible to continue any legitimate research and turned its use into an underground phenomena.

Very quickly the War on Drugs had targets that were even broader than before. Race, class, and anti-authoritarian populations all got mixed up into this rising tide of anti-drug hysteria. President Nixon's aide, John Ehrlichman, acknowledged that the War on Drugs was a tool to target and disrupt Black communities and anti-war activists. The deliberate association of drugs with minority groups aimed to vilify these communities, perpetuating stereotypes and justifying aggressive law enforcement measures.

Simultaneously, economic disparities further exacerbated the discriminatory impact of drug policies. Inner-city neighborhoods, predominantly inhabited by people of color, were disproportionately affected by economic hardships. These communities lacked adequate resources, education, and economic opportunities, leading many individuals toward illicit activities, including the drug trade. Instead of addressing the root causes of poverty and limited opportunities, the response was punitive, contributing to a cycle of criminalization that further marginalized these communities.

And then there was Ronald Reagan, who, in my opinion, made Nixon's drug policies look like they came from a moderate. At least Nixon left room for treatment centers and the establishment of federal aid to fund them. Reagan wanted none of that. The "Just Say No" era of the 1980s was dumb, void of nuance and compassion, and somehow took all the progress we made in the 1960s and threw it out the window. From a political perspective, it was like it never happened at all.

The policies enacted during Reagan's War on Drugs were characterized by even harsher penalties for drug offenses, including mandatory minimum sentences that saw racially influenced examples, like the penalties for crack cocaine becoming twenty times more severe than for the possession of powder cocaine. These clearly racially biased policies resulted in the mass incarceration of individuals predominantly from minority communities, leading to a significant increase in the prison population. On June 29, 1990, 47 percent of the US population in jails were Black men. The remaining 51 percent of the population was made up of white men and 2 percent of other races. To add an even more shocking perspective, in 1974, 8.7 percent of all adult Black men were imprisoned, and by 2001 that number doubled to 16 percent. By 2022, Black people were admitted to jail at four times the rate of white people.

And when it comes to drug-related offenses the US Justice Department itself claims, "An estimated two-thirds of those in state prisons for drug offenses were convicted of trafficking or manufacturing illegal drugs . . . Since 1985, the number of adult arrests for drug violations has increased by 74 percent and the number of arrests for sales or manufacturing of illegal drugs has grown by 137 percent." Take a moment and ponder those statistics for a minute. This is the cold, hard reality of the War on Drugs.

This reality of American life created a cycle of criminalization that perpetuated social and economic disparities as individuals with criminal records faced barriers to employment, housing, and social reintegration upon release. Furthermore, the disparities in law enforcement practices became evident through racial profiling and selective targeting. Studies consistently showed that despite similar rates of drug use across racial lines, people of color were disproportionately arrested, prosecuted, and sentenced for drug-related offenses compared to their white counterparts. This disparity reflected systemic biases within law enforcement and the criminal justice system.

The consequences of the War on Drugs continue to reverberate through society. Decades of punitive drug policies have strained resources, perpetuated cycles of poverty, and exacerbated social divisions. This is the War on Drugs: a failed experiment of policy, racial discrimination, and a propaganda campaign that has been decades long in the making. The false narratives in popular culture and education circles alone will take years to unravel and course correct.

In recent years, there has been a growing acknowledgment of the failures of the War on Drugs. Efforts to reform drug policies—including the decriminalization of certain substances, diversion programs, and a shift toward rehabilitation rather than punitive measures—have gained momentum. However, the legacy of discriminatory policies persists, necessitating comprehensive reforms that address both racial inequalities and socioeconomic disparities to achieve meaningful change in drug policy and its societal impact. Among all those recently surveyed, no matter their political party preference, 82 percent believe that the federal government should change the laws surrounding drug policies.

Polling data and public sentiment aside, this world does not exist—yet. Laws are changing before our very eyes, and our political representatives are slowly catching up to the beliefs of their constituents. We are seeing a widening shift in changing the conversation. The data does not lie.

Decriminalization and Legalization of Psychedelics

Focusing on psychedelics alone, both Colorado and Oregon have decriminalized the possession and use of magic mushrooms and are setting the stage for legal therapeutic use. At the time of writing this book, there is in fact legal access to psilocybin-assisted therapy in Oregon. The first legal sessions have taken place and, so far, show no signs of danger or further destabilization. This brings me back to the medical versus recreational use debate among the psychedelic community. Some believe that psychedelics should only be decriminalized for use in psychedelic-assisted therapy, and others believe that sacred, Indigenous, and safe recreational use should be looked at as well.

Even among our own community, there is a glitch in the matrix.

I've been to many psychedelic conferences where I've seen expert policy panelists talking about the need for very tight restrictions that allow for the use of psychedelics only under the supervision of trained psychedelic therapists, and even then, they say the use should only apply to those seeking treatment for mental health. Later on in the evening, at any of the many conference after-parties, I see the same people rolling on MDMA or eating mushroom chocolate bars. This isn't meant to shame these people or call them out; it's meant to amplify the blatant and counter-constructive hypocrisy that exists even in our community. You can't have it both ways. If the people advocating for policy changes can't even stand up for cognitive liberty and are themselves hiding in the closet as recreational psychedelic users, then I'm afraid the road is much longer than it needs to be.

One of the great advancements of the modern psychedelic movement is that it has created a safe space for many users to come out of hiding and talk about the positive effects these drugs have had on their lives. Their use is no longer relegated to counterculture-oriented psychonauts. Many business leaders, Silicon Valley titans, clergy, veterans, athletes, and medical doctors who have all been worried about what it means to publicly advocate for these drugs in the past are now attesting to their benefits. Even with that, one of the damaging ripples that the War on Drugs narrative has created is that it is somehow immoral, embarrassing, or shameful to use an illegal drug successfully. As if the admission of doing so somehow makes you less of a good citizen.

Dr. Carl Hart, the author of the book *Drug Use for Grown-Ups*, has become one of my modern-day heroes due to the very sound and plainspoken benefits that he has personally found with the use of recreational drugs that are horribly demonized in American culture. He says, "I am now entering my fifth year as a regular heroin user . . . I do not have a drug-use problem. Never have. Each day, I meet my parental, personal, and professional responsibilities. I pay my taxes, serve as a volunteer in my community on a regular basis, and contribute to the global community as an informed and engaged citizen. I am better for my drug use."

A 2020 Gallup poll puts the number of Americans who use cannabis at 12 percent. That sits roughly around 25 million to 28 million people when you subtract those underage who use this compound regularly. These are big numbers. So big that it must inform our views (both legal and social) on the incorporation of drugs for purposes other than medical.

When an illegal behavior is repeated over and over again by such a large number of people, the law that criminalizes that behavior is no longer a sound punitive one that protects our society. It is a civil war that prosecutes some people when convenient and looks the other way when not.

As I said in the beginning of this chapter, I do not have the answers. I am not a policy wonk and will be the first to admit that psychedelics aren't for everyone. Neither is alcohol, and that can be found in every street corner market in America. I tend to lean toward a solution that can allow for all voices to be heard and one where cognitive liberty remains a legitimate cause for the citizen who wants to set forth on a journey that makes sense for them and hurts no one else.

Rick Doblin, the founder of MAPS, has adopted Timothy's "driver's license" model for recreational use—one that loosely states that if you want to use a psychedelic at home and in an intentional way that you could perhaps obtain some sort of permission slip from a local mental health professional that would grant you access to buy these drugs. That's not dissimilar to the medicalized cannabis system where you go to get a medical card that allows you to walk into the smoke shop and buy the flower. That's one solution for sure. But with that comes a lot of bureaucracy and individuals who can take advantage of the system—i.e., people who feign symptoms to obtain a medical cannabis card and then go off to smoke recreationally.

Psychedelic-assisted therapy is a no-brainer, and the mental health efficacy far outweighs any risks associated with psychedelic use. As far as recreational use goes, I can't say with any sort of conviction that allowing an adult to buy a quarter ounce of mushrooms poses any more threat to our society than anything else that is legal. Alcohol, tobacco, and firearms are much more dangerous and result in far more deaths than a legal quarter ounce of mushrooms ever will.

Whatever the case is or isn't, I don't think the current legal status of psychedelics should deter you from making a decision that you feel is right for your own evolution. That sounds like I am endorsing and even encouraging illegal behavior.

"Think for yourself and question authority," Timothy Leary said, and this is probably the best advice I can give you as well. If your job, housing, or parenting rights of your children would be put at risk should you choose to go on a psychedelic journey, then you might want to consider that before doing it. But if you can find a way to explore your extraordinary and untapped inner world that doesn't endanger your livelihood, then by all means do the research and find the best way to do it safely.

The government hasn't led us to new heights in a long, long time. Governments are led by the will of the people. We cannot wait for the local authority to lead the way in granting this form of personal freedom—they will listen to you. We see this happening in the psychedelic world all the time. Politicians are waking up and realizing that psychedelics can play a huge role in treating mental health and that the War on Drugs has failed. With everything that is going on in our country today, I'd have to put the illegal use of recreational drugs, including psychedelics, toward the bottom of the list.

Education, criminal justice reform, and the rewriting of narratives around drug use will create a safer and more informed public that can make better decisions.

Afterword

Parting Thoughts, Resources, and Final Suggestions

Now that you've made it to the end of this book's journey, my hope is that you've opened your mind to the possibility that healing, personal and spiritual growth, and the exploration of different states of consciousness with the aid of psychedelic medicines is a worthwhile and legitimate method. Yoga, mindfulness, breathwork, and psychotherapy all have their place in Western culture as valuable practices for improving one's life. Yet, psychedelics still have a stigma attached to them. My intent in writing this book was to address some of that stigma by providing advice, background, and commentary on the use of these drugs in hopes that the cultural narrative can course correct itself just a little bit.

Also, some of my desire for what you've taken away from this book depends on how you came to pick it up in the first place. If you had some psychedelic experience, I hope you can continue forth on your journey of self-inquiry with some tools that may expand your knowledge base for how to use these substances even more safely and with more introspection and efficacy. The mind is a powerful thing and even the most experienced user of psychedelic drugs will continue to be surprised by the unpredictable nature of what it is to dive deeper into the nature of their own humanity with the aid of psychedelics.

If you are new to psychedelics but came in with an open mind, then perhaps you've discovered a road map for personal and therapeutic use that can help you maximize your upcoming experiences. And if you're a skeptic and are purely intellectually curious, then maybe you've resonated with some of the stories, research, and personal experiences that have been shared. Hopefully they have changed your mind, even if it's only slightly. I find that most people who are anti-psychedelics are that way due to the vast amount of propaganda and misinformation that has been disseminated for decades via media and popular culture. For instance, when I tell hardcore skeptics the stories of American veterans whose lives have been literally saved because of psychedelic treatment, their eyes widen with a shock of surprise and a "Really? Tell me more" attitude. I realize that change doesn't happen overnight, but by sharing stories of some of the most profound transformations, it can help chip away at those solid bricks of cognitive bias.

Finally, for everyone who read this book—no matter what side of the fence you are on—perhaps some of the historical context of psychedelic use, their introduction to Western culture, the War on Drugs, and some of the touching personal stories of transformation will cause you to see this movement in a different light. Since the 1960s, psychedelic drugs have changed the very tapestry of Western life in ways that are both obvious and subtle. Loud and colorful influences found in music, art, film, fashion, spirituality, and ecology are but a few of the areas touched by positive psychedelic use. Because of the persecution of drug use in America, countless people have been afraid to come out of hiding out of fear of persecution and ridicule for their trumpeting of inner transformation thanks to psychedelic use. The shifting culture of psychedelic therapy from fringe to mainstream has created more tolerance and safety for those in hiding to come out and talk about it. That change in attitude is a necessary one in every form of personal growth there is. Psychedelic use, religious affiliation, sexual or gender affiliation, and ideological leanings all require every one of us to not judge. It requires us to listen and learn tolerance in its truest form. We are living in a world that is becoming increasingly polarized and divisive. I am thankful that psychedelics have reached a larger audience, but more so, I am especially hopeful that some of the people whose minds have been changed can extend that same transformation to other parts of our society.

Some Final Suggestions

Scattered throughout the chapters of this book are some suggestions on how to better use psychedelics from both a more expansive side and a therapeutic side. However, after reading those suggestions you might be left wondering, *Okay, so now what? Where do I start?*

Many people who helped me complete this book suggested that I provide some specific recommendations on where one might look to find a psychedelic guide, for instance. After careful consideration, I decided not to include resources for that specifically. As of publication, the use of psychedelics with or without a guide is still illegal, and most people who do formal guiding are doing it underground. My main concern with that is not so much the endorsement of an illegal activity as much as a safety concern. Currently there is no one resource available that curates psychedelic guides and vouches for their safety and efficacy. The good news is that if you are curious about embarking on a fully legal psychedelic experience, there are a few exceptions that can help start your journey.

Oregon

Ballot Measure 109 was passed by Oregon voters in 2020 and allows psilocybin to be used legally under the supervision of licensed therapeutic professionals. You can start your journey by visiting the Oregon State website. There, you can find licensed facilitators and healing centers. When visiting the site, think of it as visiting *Psychology Today* or something of that nature. Look for someone who resonates with you and what is it you are after.

Religious Freedom Act (Psychedelic Churches)

The Native American Church (NAC) was granted legal use of peyote for religious purposes in the United States with the passage of the American Indian Religious Freedom Act (AIRFA) in 1978. This legislation affirmed the right of Native Americans to practice their traditional spiritual beliefs, including the sacramental use of peyote, a cactus containing the psychoactive compound mescaline. The use of peyote in religious ceremonies predates the establishment of the NAC and has deep roots in various Native American cultures. The legal protection provided by AIRFA was further strengthened by subsequent amendments and court rulings to safeguard the religious rights of Native Americans to use peyote as a sacrament in their ceremonies.

This was a landmark ruling in the Indigenous use of psychedelics in America. More recently, many others who are of nonindigenous persuasions have used the Religious Freedom Act as a way to grant legal and ceremonial use of psychedelics as sacraments. Many have taken advantage of these laws and used them merely as a legal loophole, while others do indeed treat these substances with tremendous respect and hold them in high integrity.

While still illegal on a federal level, these churches are walking a line legally, but in my opinion, they are doing it within an acceptable legal protection. There are many scattered throughout the country that you can find with a simple Google search, but, as mentioned, not all are reputable. Please do your research on which ones are serving these medicines with an aim of safety and ritual and not increased profits.

I hold great respect for David Hodges, chief priest at the Church of Ambrosia in Oakland, California, who has the largest psilocybin membership church in the world (over 90,000 members at the time of writing this). And in the states Texas and Colorado the ATMA Church and Ceremonia are both legal churches that serve various psychedelics with great care and integrity.

Psychedelic Tourism

Psychedelic tourism is a vast and expansive industry with popularity in countries where certain psychedelics are legal. Ayahuasca is legal for ceremonial use in Peru and Brazil, for instance, and there are many wonderful retreat centers to visit should you want to take that journey.

While I can't provide real-time browsing or endorse specific websites, there are reputable resources available online that can help you find information on Ayahuasca retreat centers in Peru. Here are some general tips and suggestions on how to find reliable information:

1. **Research Ayahuasca communities:** Look for online forums, communities, or social media groups dedicated to Ayahuasca and plant medicine. These platforms often have discussions, reviews, and recommendations from individuals who have experienced various retreat centers firsthand.

2. **Consult Ayahuasca retreat directories:** There are websites dedicated to listing Ayahuasca retreat centers, such as Ayamundo, AyaAdvisors, and Retreat Guru. These directories provide information on different centers, including their location, offerings, reviews, and ratings from past participants.

3. **Check reviews and testimonials:** Look for reviews and testimonials from people who have attended Ayahuasca retreats. However, it's essential to critically evaluate the credibility of reviews and consider a range of opinions.

4. **Contact retreat centers directly:** Once you've narrowed down your options, consider reaching out to the retreat centers directly. Ask questions about their facilitators, safety protocols, accommodations, and the overall structure of their programs.

5. **Verify credentials and legal compliance:** Ensure that the retreat center and its facilitators have the necessary credentials, such as training in shamanism or traditional healing practices. Additionally, verify that the center operates legally and adheres to local regulations regarding Ayahuasca ceremonies.

6. **Trust your intuition:** Ultimately, trust your instincts and intuition when selecting an Ayahuasca retreat center. Pay attention to how you feel about the center's philosophy, atmosphere, and the people involved.

Remember that participating in an Ayahuasca retreat is a deeply personal and potentially transformative experience. It's crucial to approach it with caution, respect, and thorough research to ensure your safety and well-being. Additionally, always consult with health-care professionals before participating in ceremonies, especially if you have underlying medical conditions or are taking medications.

Psychedelic Integration Coaches

While psychedelics aren't legal to use with an underground guide, it is 100 percent legal to seek and hire a psychedelic integration coach for after your journey. Many of those you'll find on the following listing services have gone through some form of training or are licensed mental health professionals. The same rules apply in finding someone to help you with this aspect of the process. Not everyone listed is suited for you, so do your homework, schedule a consult call, and take the time to find the person that is right for you and your specific desires. Some good resources are Psychedelic.support, Thethirdwave.co, Trippingly.net, Psycle.clinic, and Being True To You.

Community

In some ways, having community support is the most important recommendation I can make. My father famously said, "Find the others," and that couldn't be more useful when entering the world of psychedelics. Going at it alone is a risky proposition. The more you gather in community and talk to experts and people who have been through it, the more informed and better off you'll be. In nearly every major city in the Western world, there is a local psychedelic society that gathers regularly to provide talks, panels, and integration circles. Many of them are extremely well organized and very well attended. They are beautiful testaments to the power of community and the inspired nature of wanting to share your psychedelic breakthroughs with others. No matter what stage of the journey you are on, I highly recommend that you plug in to your local psychedelic society to learn, grow, share, and gather.

This is one aspect of psychedelic use that many Indigenous communities have baked into their culture that we have not. They have generations upon generations of family and neighbors that have spent time with these medicines and can act as a buffer upon returning from ceremony. Western society, for the most part, does not have this communal relationship with psychedelic drugs. That is slowly changing as more and more people feel safe enough to come out of the psychedelic closet, but there are still miles to go.

Rather than providing some recommendations, there is one overarching body that (sort of) governs all local chapters. It's more of an egalitarian approach than it is a governmental one, meaning they are all free to assemble in any style or format they want as long as they maintain safety. The Global Psychedelic Society website provides listings for nearly all of the psychedelic communities around the world.

Go forward with rabid curiosity, an open mind, and an air of cautious optimism. The road of spiritual, mental, and cognitive healing with the aid of psychedelics is vast and sometimes scary. I encourage you to listen to that deepest part of your intuition as you determine if these drugs are right for you. Others may inspire you, but only you can think for yourself.

Acknowledgments

For anyone who is about to write their first book, I want to briefly share a little of my story behind the creation of this one. It leads into why it's so important that I stop and thank the people who were mission critical in helping make this book a reality.

Prior to writing the book, I went through a dark night of the soul and now I see clearly that this offering is a representation of the hope and love that I received now that the dark night turned to a beautiful morning. I am healthy, happy, and very proud of what I've created.

In 2020, I had the idea for the book in a slightly different form, and took it upon myself to write the book proposal. I did that in three days. Over forty pages came to me in a graceful download of thought and words in what seemed like an instant. It was magic! Not long after that, I was lucky enough to find a home for the idea at Sounds True. Because that portion of the project happened so quickly, I thought to myself, *Wow. This is easy. I'll have the book done in nine months.* That was not the case. The proposal was indeed a gift from the heavens, but the hard work that it took to complete the manuscript took much longer than I thought it would. Missed deadlines, inspirational struggles, scattered processes, and a loss of hope scared me. The book finally did come to fruition after I once again dug deep and simply chopped wood and carried water. It was the hardest thing I've ever had to do in my life. But I am happy to report back that the crazy process did help me learn how to do something new. Should I choose to do it again, I'll look back on this as my larval phase.

On the dedication page I, without hesitation, dedicated this book to my father Timothy and to my mentor and teacher Ram Dass. Without them I would not be the person I am today. Not only did they give me a once-in-a-lifetime front row seat to the subject material of this book, but they also gifted me a method for finding my own voice that I'm not so sure I would have found had they not been there for me. Their impact on my life is unmeasurable.

After that, my partner Heather is the person I'd like to thank most for making this possible. After the aforementioned dark night of the soul, Heather and I rekindled our partnership and found an even deeper connection of trust, love, and being each other's biggest fans. The safety and sheer act of being seen by her allowed me to write this book in a way that made sense for my nonlinear process—free from judgment or scorn, just love. So Heather, thank you. I couldn't have done it without you.

The problem with an acknowledgment section of any project is that I'm sure I will forget a few people by name, but here are some essential others who have played a huge part in my life and in this book.

Jennifer Brown and Sarah Stanton at Sounds True for your patience and guidance as I stumbled through this process. And Tami Simon for creating such a rich legacy that I am proud to be a part of.

Gretel Hakanson for helping edit and streamline this into something better than it was. Your work on this book helped me see where I made mistakes and how to improve upon them.

Cesar, Liz, and Ted; Bruce L., Craig, and Mariasha P.W.; Ron M., John B. of my recovery community for never giving up on me.

Shiva, Narayan, Amy, Zoe, Govind Das, Krishna Das, ShyamDas, Dasi Ma, Mike Crall, Jack and Trudy, Mirabai, and so many others in the Bhakti and Ram Dass satsang whose light may not be currently near but is always in my heart.

John and Patrick Baker, Sean Colgin, and Gary for keeping me a part of the longest Dodgers text thread ever, which has helped keep me grounded and sane over the years.

Hal, Chris, Dana—my brothers and friends no matter what.

To the people at MAPS, past and present, who let me run with the podcast—Rick Doblin, Bryce Montgomery, Matt Neal, Betty Aldworth, Whitney, and Christine. Hosting the podcast gave me insight into a fantastic, brave, new world of psychedelic research and culture.

Terence and Denis McKenna, Albert Hofmann, Alan Watts, Sasha and Ann Shulgin, Dr. John C. Lilly, Ralph Metzner, Marina Sabina, Stan Grof, Aldous and Laura Huxley—to name but a few from the first phase of Western psychedelic thinkers who helped blow this movement wide open by creating an entirely new paradigm for people like me to explore their consciousness. I am so fortunate to have known some of them in my younger years, and their humility and authentic curiosity is something I'll never forget.

Every listener of my podcast, every student who has taken my course, and every person who has sent me a loving email of support—those go such a long way, you have no idea how much.

And of course my mother, Barbara, who has been my teacher, friend, and wonderful mother throughout all the ups and downs in life. I love you.

And finally, Neem Karoli Baba and the Grateful Dead for showing the path of grace. Ram ram.

Index

loving awareness, 123

LSD, 11, 39–44
  clinical studies, 24, 68
  folklorish history, 42
  Hofmann, Albert, 40, 42
  questions to ask yourself before an
    LSD journey, 44
  treatment for alcohol addiction,
    153–54

MAOIs (monoamine oxidase inhibitors),
  33
Maté, Gabor, 87–88, 150
McKenna, Terence, 29, 52–53, 58, 101
MDMA, 13, 22, 32, 45–48, 65–68
  PTSD treatment, 65–67, 77–80,
    90–95, 176–77
  questions to ask yourself before an
    MDMA journey, 47–48
medicalization model, 62–63
  moving toward a successful model,
    82–83
  pros and cons, 72–76
meditation, 26, 109, 142, 186, 199
Metzner, Ralph, 22
MK-ULTRA, 40
monkey mind, 109–12
Multidisciplinary Association for
  Psychedelic Studies (MAPS), 12–13,
  41, 65–68, 77–80, 90, 93–94
mushrooms. *See* psilocybin

Native American Church, 59, 220
neuroplasticity, 24

Nixon, Richard, 10, 12, 42, 209–10
Nova, Danielle, 155–56, 160

"the one," 110
Osmond, Humphry, 7, 41, 153

Pollan, Michael, 28, 69, 127
psilocybin, 6, 25, 27, 34, 48–50
  author's use of, 151–53
  Compass Pathways and synthesizing
    psilocybin-like compounds, 70–71
  decriminalization, 212, 219
  depression, 34
  end-of-life anxiety, 167–69
  neuroplasticity, 24
  "Not So Fast on Psychedelic
    Mushrooms" (*New York Times*
    op-ed), 69
  personal account of healing effects,
    96–97
  questions to ask yourself before a
    psilocybin journey, 50
psychedelic churches, 220
The Psychedelic Experience (Leary,
  Metzner, and Alpert), 70, 164,
  173–74
psychedelic experience, 27–35
  dissolution of boundaries, 29–30
  emotional resonance, 31
  expanded states of consciousness,
    30–31
  hallucinatory visions and space-time
    dissolution, 30
psychedelic renaissance, 5
psychedelic tourism, 221–22

About the Author

Over the course of the last thirty years, Zach has found himself in the center of the psychedelic movement with a front row seat to the modern renaissance while also having firsthand knowledge of the historical legacy of the counterculture's influence on psychedelic exploration.

After spending many years as a digital marketing expert for some of the world's largest brands, Zach had a wakeup call thirteen years ago that thrust him back into the center of the psychedelic cyclone, thanks to the influence of his primary teacher and mentor, Ram Dass. Since then, he has found his own unique voice and method in being able to contribute to the revolutionary new psychedelic movement of the twenty-first century.

As a health and wellness facilitator, integration coach, session guide, podcaster, writer, and seeker of all things mystical, Zach has worked with nearly two hundred people one on one to help them heal with the assistance of psychedelic medicines. And as a teacher, Zach has taught over one hundred people his unique approach to psychedelic studies, safe use and harm reduction, the history of psychedelics, and how to be a well-rounded, knowledgeable, and safe practitioner.

Zach currently hosts the *Psychedelics Then and Now* podcast, has in-depth knowledge of psychedelic-assisted facilitation, and is a trained meditation teacher, a student of bhakti yoga, an IFS enthusiast, and an expert in the history of psychedelic culture and its many methodologies.

Zach is also an avid musician, a kirtan singer, and a still-practicing Deadhead.

About Sounds True

Sounds True was founded in 1985 by Tami Simon with a clear mission: to disseminate spiritual wisdom. Since starting out as a project with one woman and her tape recorder, we have grown into a multimedia publishing company with a catalog of more than 3,000 titles by some of the leading teachers and visionaries of our time, and an ever-expanding family of beloved customers from across the world.

In more than three decades of evolution, Sounds True has maintained our focus on our overriding purpose and mission: to wake up the world. We offer books, audio programs, online learning experiences, and in-person events to support your personal growth and awakening, and to unlock our greatest human capacities to love and serve.

At SoundsTrue.com you'll find a wealth of resources to enrich your journey, including our weekly *Insights at the Edge* podcast, free downloads, and information about our nonprofit Sounds True Foundation, where we strive to remove financial barriers to the materials we publish through scholarships and donations worldwide.

To learn more, please visit SoundsTrue.com/freegifts or call us toll-free at 800.333.9185.

Together, we can wake up the world.

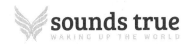